# *AN ATLAS of* ___

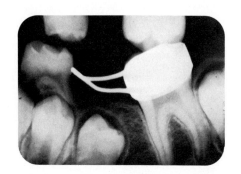 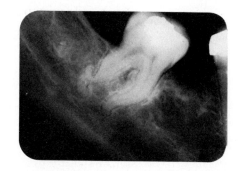

# DENTAL RADIOGRAPHIC ANATOMY

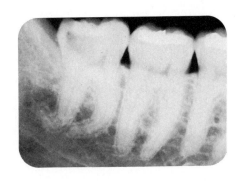

MYRON J. KASLE, D.D.S., M.S.D.

CHAIRMAN,
Department of Dental Radiology
Indiana University School of Dentistry
Indianapolis, Indiana

SECOND EDITION

1983
W. B. SAUNDERS COMPANY
Philadelphia, London, Toronto, Mexico City, Rio de Janeiro, Sydney, Tokyo

W. B. Saunders Company:  West Washington Square
Philadelphia, PA  19105

1 St. Anne's Road
Eastbourne, East Sussex BN21 3UN, England

1 Goldthorne Avenue
Toronto, Ontario M8Z 5T9, Canada

Apartado 26370—Cedro 512
Mexico 4, D.F., Mexico

Rua Coronel Cabrita, 8
Sao Cristovao Caixa Postal 21176
Rio de Janeiro, Brazil

9 Waltham Street
Artarmon, N.S.W. 2064, Australia

Ichibancho, Central Bldg., 22-1 Ichibancho
Chiyoda-Ku, Tokyo 102, Japan

Listed here are the latest translated editions of this book together
with the language of the translation and the publisher.

French (*1st Edition*)—Masson Editeur Paris, France

Japanese (*1st Edition*)—The Shorin Company Ltd., Tokyo, Japan

Portuguese (*1st Edition*)—Editora Interamericana Ltda. Rio de Janeiro, Brazil

An Atlas of Dental Radiographic Anatomy          ISBN  0-7216-1036-6

Last digit is the print number:     9     8     7     6     5     4     3     2     1

*TO MY WIFE, JUDY,*
*AND TO MY SONS, MICHAEL AND RICHARD*

# *Foreword*

In the field of dental radiology we are continuing to witness a revitalization of interest in the intraoral and extraoral techniques, as well as in the interpretation of high quality films. Two of the reasons for this renewal of interest are the increasing importance attached to the need for complete preoperative records and the realization that accurate and thorough interpretation of radiographs is essential to the development of a comprehensive treatment plan for the dental patient.

Dr. Kasle's well-received *Atlas of Dental Radiographic Anatomy* is now available in this second, expanded edition. If this Atlas is studied in a careful and systematic manner, the reader will be provided with an excellent review of anatomic landmarks. It is possible for the reader to open the book to almost any page and in a few minutes be reminded of important observations that affect treatment planning in dental practice.

The second edition offers additional material on temporomandibular joint radiographs and accompanying case reports. There is a renewed interest in this topic, including the degenerative changes that are often seen in this anatomical region. The new edition also includes illustrations of many common errors in radiographic technique, including faulty placement of film, processing errors, and film artifacts. Special attention to the avoidance of these common errors will reduce the need for retakes and additional patient radiation exposure. A careful study of the book will also serve as a review of successful and unsuccessful clinical procedures and as a refresher course in commonly observed oral pathologic conditions.

This Atlas will be a valuable addition to the library of dental practitioners and dental auxiliaries. It will be especially useful to the dental student who is becoming acquainted with the difficult task of learning radiographic interpretation.

The second edition of this outstanding book is an unusually fine and unique contribution to dentistry and specifically to effective radiographic interpretation and utilization.

Ralph E. McDonald, D.D.S.
Dean
Indiana University
School of Dentistry

# *Preface and Acknowledgements*

It is with a great deal of pleasure that the second edition of this Atlas is presented. Its acceptance by dental educators, dental students, hygiene and assisting students, and dental personnel in general has been most gratifying. The encouragement of students, present and past, has been the impetus for adding new sections to this new edition.

The intent of this Atlas is to aid the reader in relating images that are viewed on the actual clinical radiograph with those seen on the printed page. Repetition of images is necessary since individual variations are common. The reader can cover the printed page while viewing the picture, thus testing his or her knowledge of the images, which are identified with a letter.

There have been several temporomandibular joint plates, as well as two new sections, added to this edition. Since this is an Atlas, it is pictorial in nature and thus no attempt is made to explain the technical or physical principles of radiology. It is hoped that this Atlas will broaden the knowledge of all those who use it.

I wish to thank Carol Ann Steinmetz, for typing the manuscript, and Gail Williamson, L.D.H., and Dr. Jack Schaaf, faculty members in the Radiology Department, for their cooperation. Dr. Anoop Sondhi, Professor of Orthodontics at Indiana University School of Dentistry, graciously allowed me to use the films in Plates 73 to 75. Dr. James Green, University of Nebraska School of Dentistry, generously provided the materials for Plates 76 to 79.

Excellent photographic materials were again produced by Richard Scott, Director of the Illustrations Department at Indiana University School of Dentistry, and his staff, consisting of Michael Halloran and Alana Fears.

Seldom mentioned are those individuals who represent the publishers. Robert (Sandy) Reinhardt, Dental Editor, and Ray Kersey, Assistant Dental Editor for W. B. Saunders, along with a fine staff of co-workers, have all made it a pleasure to produce this volume. Their standards of quality and sensitivity to the author's needs are greatly appreciated.

I certainly cannot forget the original encouragement and advice provided by Carroll C. Cann of W. B. Saunders, when the first edition was conceived. Professor Ralph Phillips and Dean Ralph McDonald, of Indiana University School of Dentistry, have also been sources of inspiration and encouragement.

# Contents

# CONTENTS

# CONTENTS

# section one

## INTRAORAL RADIOGRAPHS

Plate 1    MAXILLARY MOLAR REGION VIEW _____

A.    Maxillary tuberosity
B.    Floor of maxillary sinus
C.    Zygomatic process
D.    Maxillary sinus
E.    Zygomatic arch
F.    Shadow of soft tissue
G.    Film identification dot
H.    Coronoid process of mandible
I.    Alveolar ridge
J.    Retained roots
K.    Pterygoid plate
L.    Palatal root of permanent second molar
M.    Mesiobuccal root of permanent first molar
N.    Overlapping of tooth contacts
O.    Floor of nasal fossa
P.    Septum in maxillary sinus
Q.    Hamulus or hamular process
R.    Groove in maxillary sinus wall for superior alveolar nerve and vessels
S.    Microdont
T.    Distal surface of permanent second bicuspid
U.    Artifact caused by fixer contamination

# PART 1 INTRAORAL RADIOGRAPHIC ANATOMY OF THE HUMAN MAXILLARY ARCH

## Plate 1 MAXILLARY MOLAR REGION VIEW

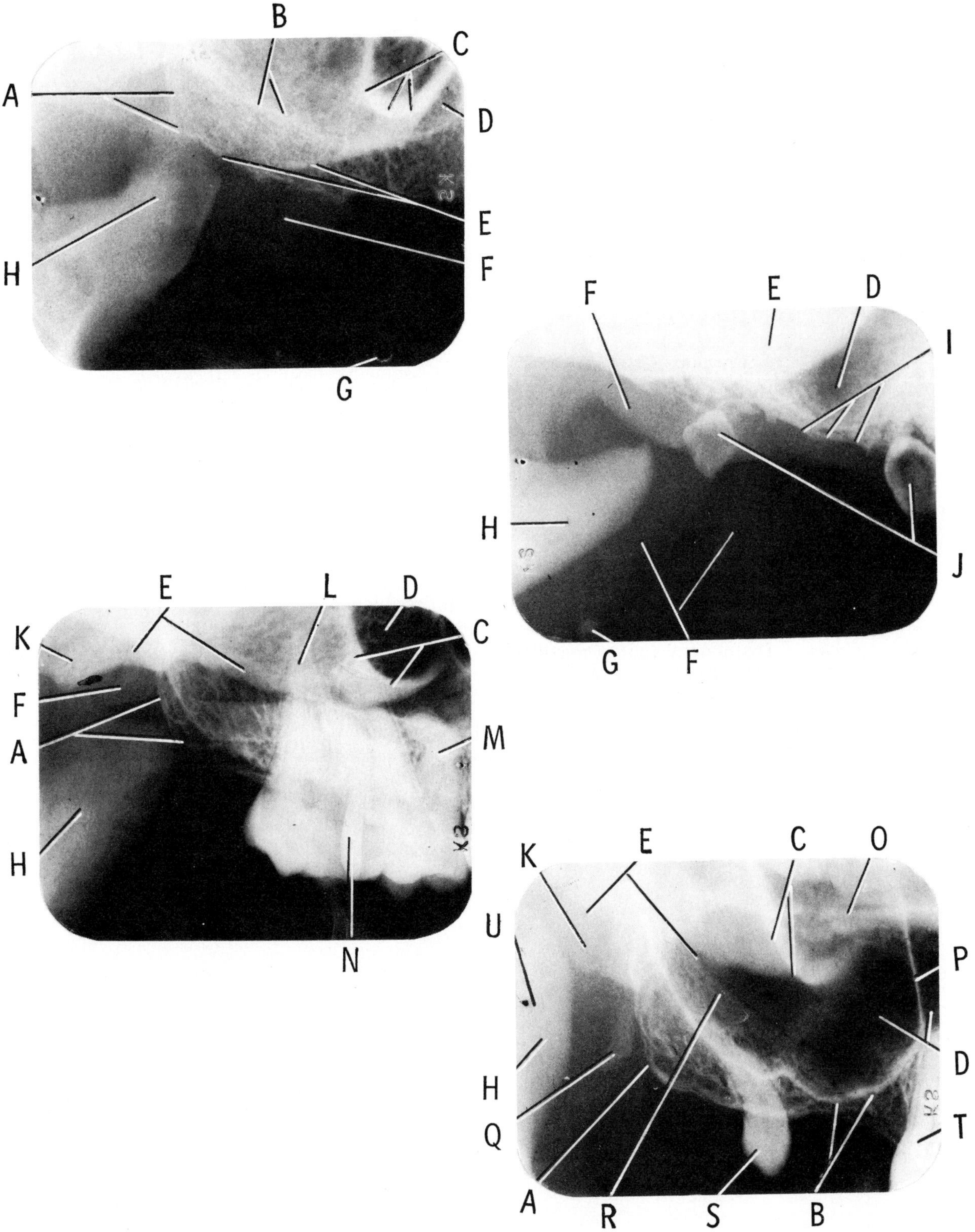

Plate 2     MAXILLARY MOLAR REGION VIEW _____

A.  Zygomatic process
B.  Maxillary sinus
C.  Posterior wall of maxillary sinus
D.  Hamular notch
E.  Maxillary tuberosity
F.  Coronoid process of mandible
G.  Lower border of zygomatic arch
H.  Palatal root of maxillary permanent first bicuspid
I.  Buccal root of maxillary permanent first bicuspid
J.  Distobuccal root of maxillary permanent first molar
K.  Mesiobuccal root of maxillary permanent first molar
L.  Dilacerated root of maxillary permanent second bicuspid
M.  Periapical radiolucency of maxillary permanent bicuspid
N.  Periapical radiolucency and buccal bone resorption of maxillary permanent first molar

Plate 2    MAXILLARY MOLAR REGION VIEW

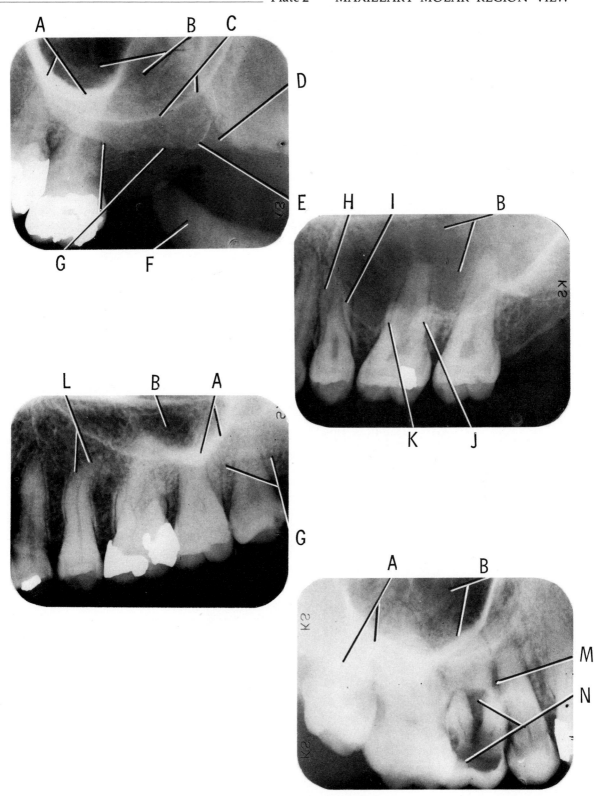

Plate 3    MAXILLARY MOLAR REGION VIEW _____

A.    Coronoid process of mandible
B.    Microdont
C.    Healed extraction site
D.    Maxillary sinus
E.    Unerupted maxillary permanent third molar
F.    Follicle of maxillary permanent third molar
G.    Hamulus — medial pterygoid plate
H.    Zygomatic process

Plate 3    MAXILLARY MOLAR REGION VIEW

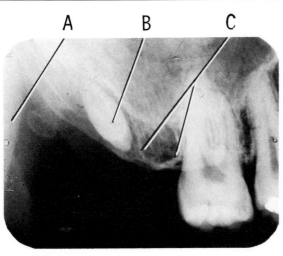

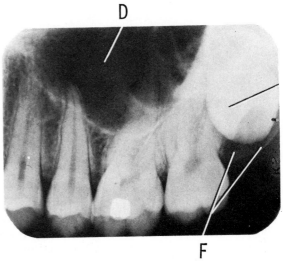

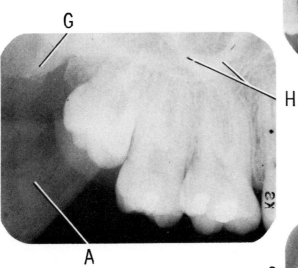

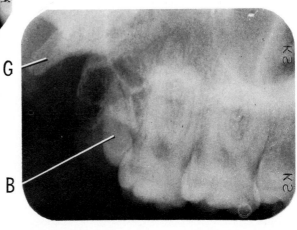

Plate 4    MAXILLARY MOLAR REGION VIEW _____

A.    Lower border of zygomatic arch
B.    Maxillary sinus
C.    Maxillary tuberosity
D.    Sclerotic bone
E.    Maxillary sinus depression
F.    Zygomatic process
G.    Lateral pterygoid plate
H.    Hamulus—medial pterygoid plate
I.    Coronoid process of mandible
J.    Film identification dot
K.    Floor of maxillary sinus
L.    Nutrient canal in maxillary sinus wall
M.    Soft tissue covering maxillary tuberosity
N.    Sequestrum from previous extraction

Plate 4    MAXILLARY MOLAR REGION VIEW

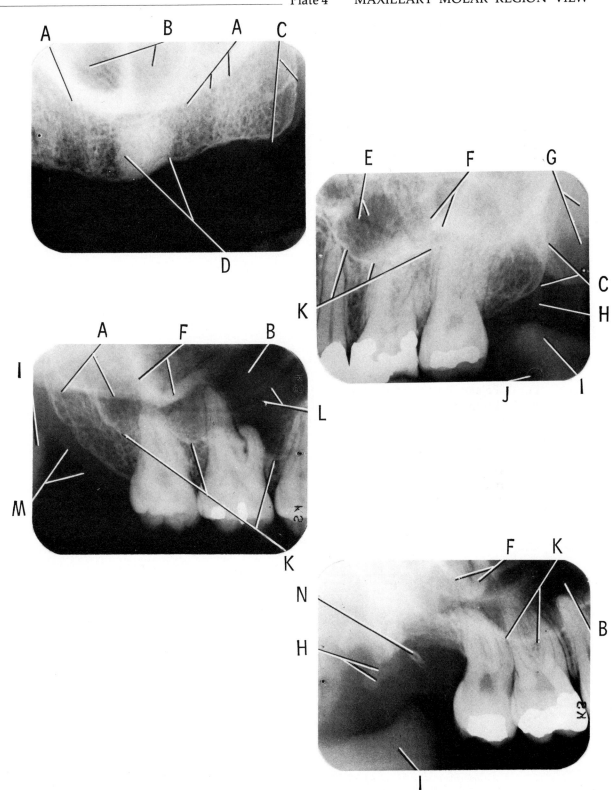

Plate 5      MAXILLARY MOLAR REGION VIEW _____

A.      Nasal fossa
B.      Floor of nasal fossa
C.      Maxillary sinus
D.      Floor of maxillary sinus
E.      Mesiobuccal root of maxillary permanent first molar
F.      Distobuccal root of maxillary permanent first molar
G.      Palatal root of maxillary permanent first molar
H.      Endodontic treatment in root of maxillary permanent second bicuspid
I.      Recurrent caries under gold crown of maxillary permanent first molar
J.      Coronoid process of mandible
K.      Film identification dot
L.      Zygomatic process
M.      Nutrient canal in maxillary sinus wall

Plate 5    MAXILLARY MOLAR REGION VIEW

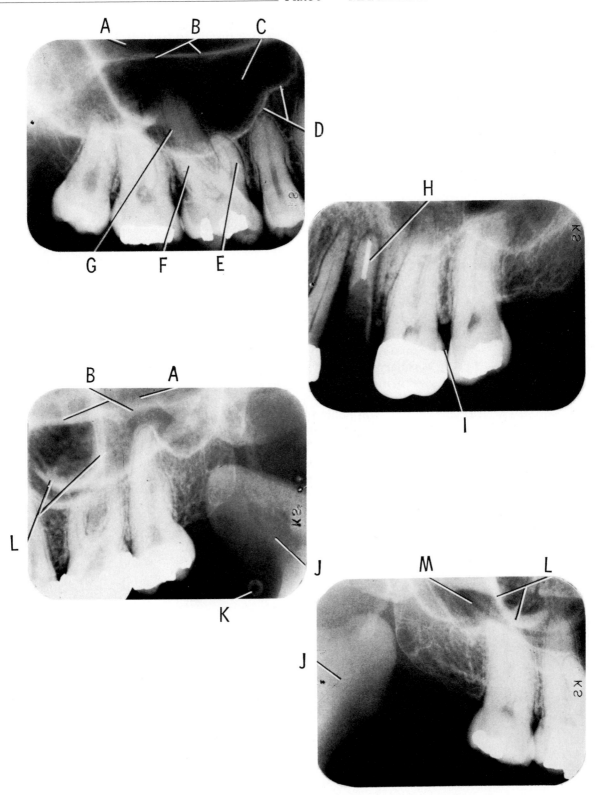

Plate 6    MAXILLARY MOLAR REGION VIEW _____

A.    Lateral pterygoid plate
B.    Hamulus—medial pterygoid plate
C.    Film identification dot
D.    Coronoid process of mandible
E.    Maxillary sinus
F.    Zygomatic process
G.    Soft tissue shadow
H.    Thin plate of bone distal to maxillary third molar
I.    Impacted maxillary permanent third molar
J.    Soft tissue over maxillary third molar
K.    Impacted supernumerary molar
L.    Chrome steel orthodontic band

Plate 6     MAXILLARY MOLAR REGION VIEW

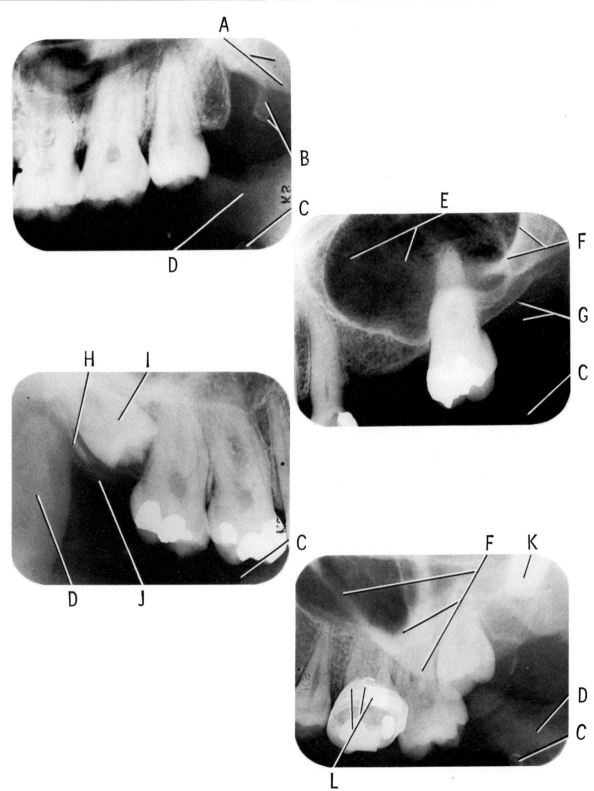

Plate 7    MAXILLARY BICUSPID REGION VIEW _____

A.   Unerupted maxillary permanent first molar
B.   Unerupted maxillary permanent second bicuspid
C.   Unerupted maxillary permanent first bicuspid
D.   Unerupted maxillary permanent cuspid
E.   Partially resorbed root of maxillary primary cuspid
F.   Maxillary primary first molar
G.   Maxillary primary second molar
H.   Radiolucent resin restoration
I.   Radiopaque metallic lingual restoration
J.   Endodontically treated maxillary permanent first bicuspid with retrograde metal restoration
K.   Gold post and core restoration
L.   Floor of nasal fossa
M.   Buccal root of maxillary permanent first bicuspid
N.   Palatal root of maxillary permanent first bicuspid
O.   Nutrient canal in maxillary sinus wall

Plate 7    MAXILLARY BICUSPID REGION VIEW

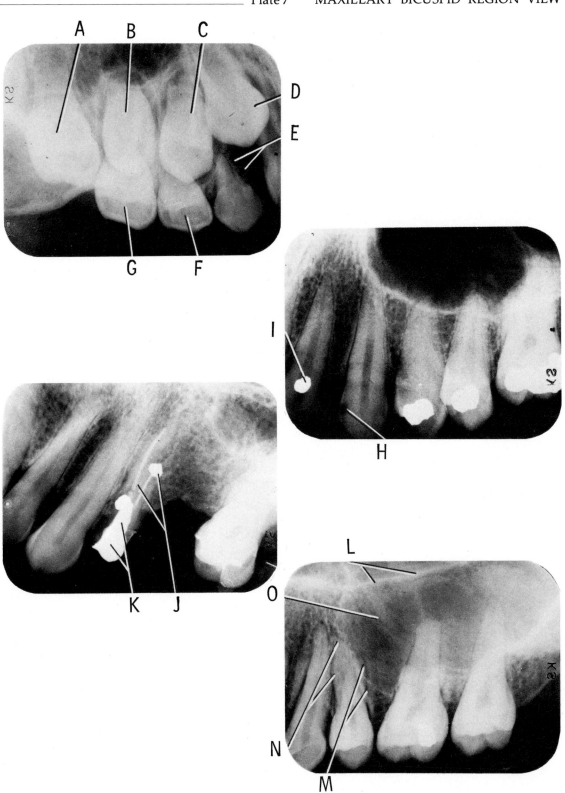

Plate 8    MAXILLARY BICUSPID REGION VIEW _____

A.    Zygomatic process
B.    Maxillary sinus
C.    Oroantral fistula
D.    Supernumerary tooth
E.    Film crease
F.    Septum in maxillary sinus
G.    Sclerosed pulp chambers
H.    Resorbed bone of edentulous arch
I.    Floor of nasal fossa
J.    Cusp of mandibular permanent first molar
K.    Maxillary primary second molar
L.    Maxillary primary first molar
M.    Maxillary primary cuspid

Plate 8     MAXILLARY  BICUSPID  REGION  VIEW

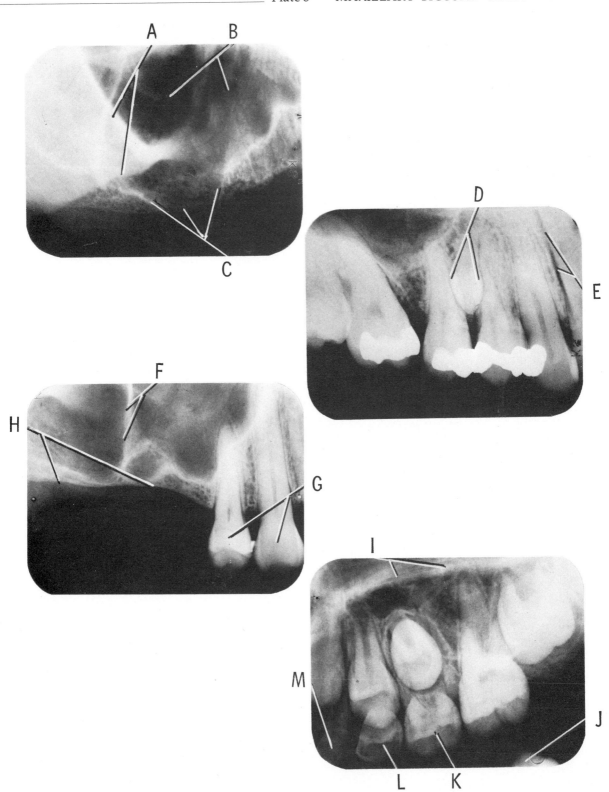

Plate 9     MAXILLARY BICUSPID REGION VIEW _____

A.     Maxillary sinus
B.     Zygoma
C.     Groove of nutrient canal in maxillary sinus
D.     Remnant of retained root tip
E.     Cervical burnout (adumbration)
F.     Septum in maxillary sinus
G.     Nasolabial fold
H.     Microdont
I.     Gold pontics
J.     Gold crown abutments

Plate 9    MAXILLARY BICUSPID REGION VIEW

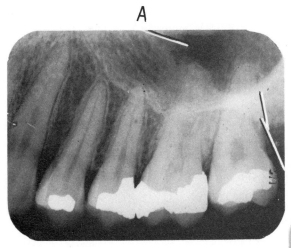

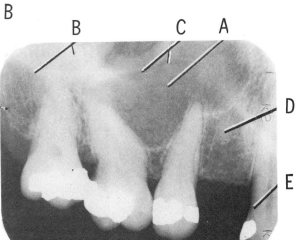

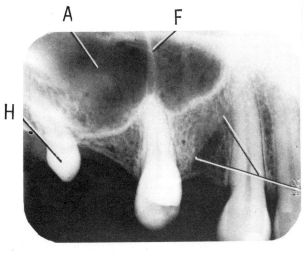

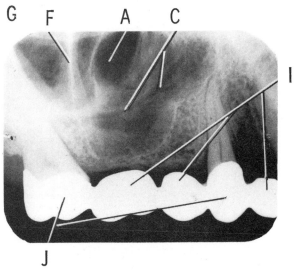

Plate 10    MAXILLARY BICUSPID REGION VIEW _____

A.    Floor of maxillary sinus
B.    Maxillary sinus
C.    Zygomatic process
D.    Carious lesions
E.    Septa in maxillary sinus
F.    Palatal root of maxillary permanent first molar
G.    Lower border of zygomatic arch
H.    Periapical radiolucency of mesial root, maxillary permanent first molar
I.    Gold crown abutment of maxillary permanent cuspid
J.    Gold pontics for maxillary bridge
K.    Gold crown abutment of maxillary permanent first molar
L.    Floor of nasal fossa

Plate 10    MAXILLARY BICUSPID REGION VIEW

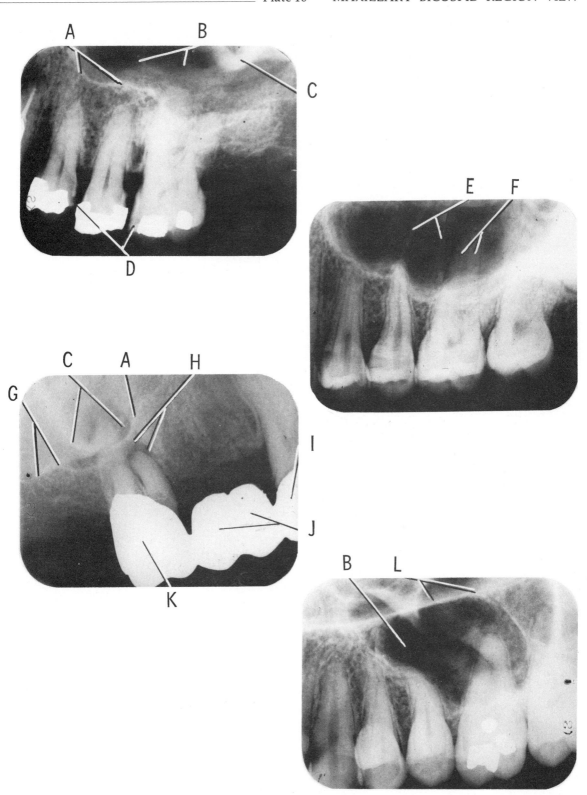

Plate 11     MAXILLARY BICUSPID–MOLAR REGION VIEW _____

A.    Maxillary sinus septum
B.    Palatal roots
C.    Maxillary tuberosity
D.    Area of bone resorption
E.    Heavy calculous deposits
F.    Compound odontoma
G.    Palatal cusp of maxillary permanent first bicuspid

Plate 11    MAXILLARY BICUSPID–MOLAR REGION VIEW

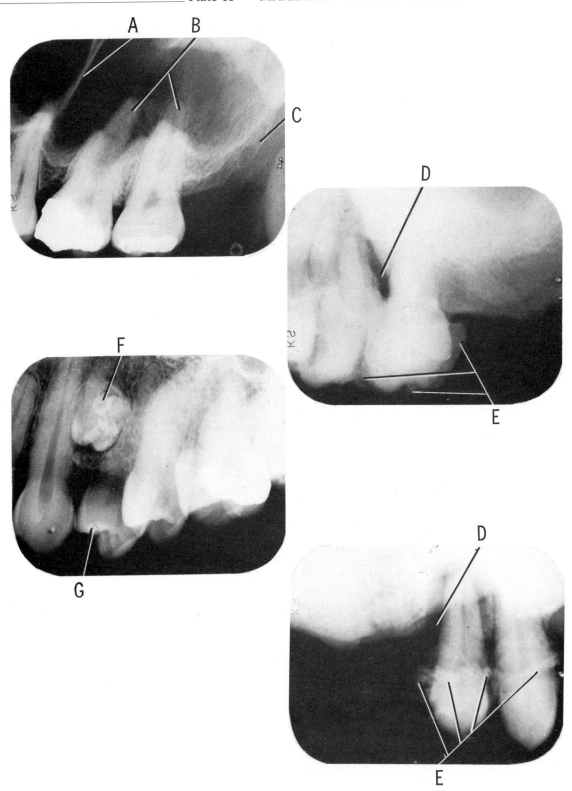

Plate 12     MAXILLARY CUSPID REGION VIEW _____

A.     Maxillary sinus
B.     Bone septum separating nasal fossa and maxillary sinus
C.     Nasal fossa
D.     Nasolabial fold
E.     Shadow of nose
F.     Cement base
G.     Resin restoration
H.     Gold post and core in endodontically treated tooth
I.     Periapical radiolucency in infected tooth
J.     Pulpally exposed tooth

Plate 12      MAXILLARY CUSPID REGION VIEW

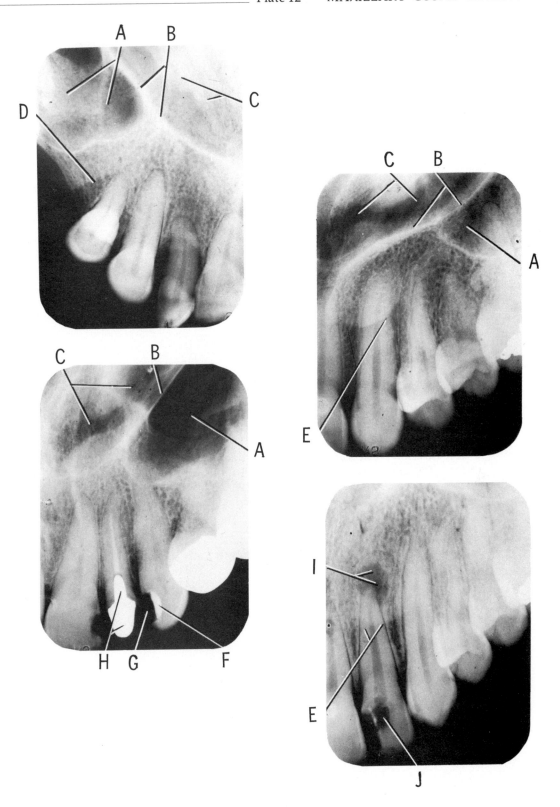

Plate 13    MAXILLARY CUSPID REGION VIEW _____

A.    Maxillary sinus
B.    Bone septum between nasal fossa and maxillary sinus
C.    Nasal fossa
D.    Radiolucent resin restorations
E.    Maxillary primary cuspid
F.    Maxillary primary first molar
G.    Nasal septum
H.    Carious lesion in maxillary permanent first bicuspid
I.    Radiopaque cement
J.    Crown prepared for jacket crown restoration
K.    Metal tubing post placed in pulp canal
L.    Carious lesion in maxillary permanent central incisor
M.    Periapical lesion due to metal tubing in pulp canal

Plate 13     MAXILLARY CUSPID REGION VIEW

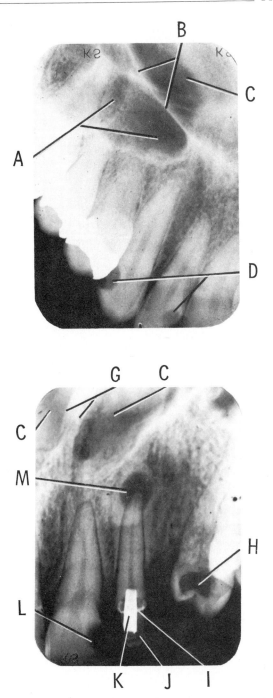

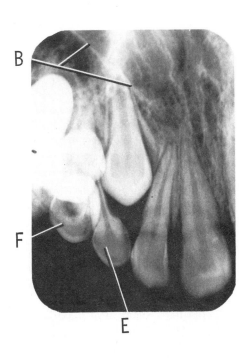

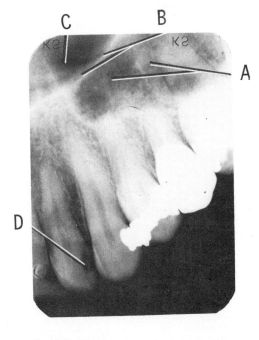

Plate 14    MAXILLARY CUSPID REGION VIEW _____

A.  Bone separating nasal fossa and maxillary sinus
B.  Nasal fossa
C.  Alveolus of recently extracted maxillary permanent lateral incisor
D.  Alveolus of recently extracted maxillary permanent central incisor
E.  Maxillary permanent cuspid
F.  Buccal cusp of maxillary permanent first bicuspid
G.  Palatal cusp of maxillary permanent first bicuspid
H.  Maxillary permanent second bicuspid
I.  Shadow of soft tissue of nose
J.  Floor of maxillary sinus
K.  Maxillary sinus
L.  Maxillary permanent central incisors
M.  Transposed maxillary permanent first bicuspid
N.  Transposed maxillary permanent cuspid
O.  Metal restorations
P.  Follicle of maxillary permanent cuspid
Q.  Incisive foramen
R.  Unerupted maxillary permanent cuspid
S.  Maxillary permanent lateral incisor
T.  Palatal cusp of maxillary permanent second bicuspid
U.  Buccal cusp of maxillary permanent second bicuspid
V.  Shadow of maxillary permanent first molar
W.  Septum in maxillary sinus
X.  Resin restorations
Y.  Film identification dot

Plate 14    MAXILLARY CUSPID REGION VIEW

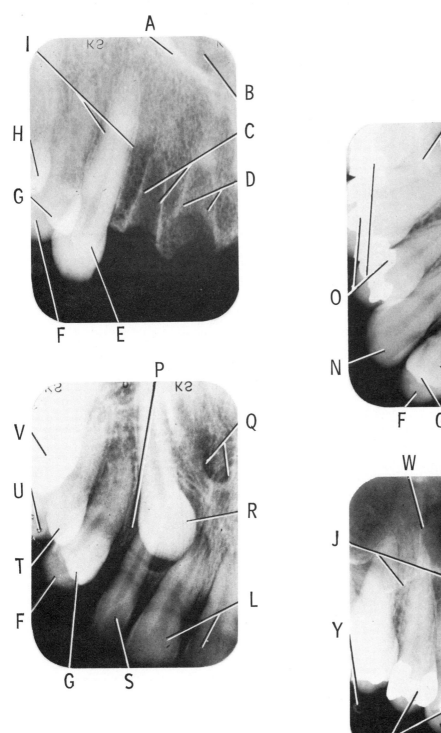

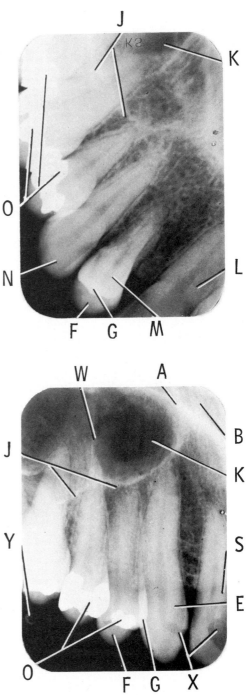

Plate 15     MAXILLARY CUSPID REGION VIEW _____

A.    Nasal fossa
B.    Floor of nasal fossa
C.    Maxillary sinus
D.    Floor of maxillary sinus
E.    Buccal root of maxillary permanent first bicuspid
F.    Palatal root of maxillary permanent first bicuspid
G.    Buccal cusp of maxillary permanent first bicuspid
H.    Resin restoration
I.    Cement base
J.    Metallic lingual restoration
K.    Film identification dot
L.    Shadow of maxillary permanent first bicuspid
M.    Overlapping contacts
N.    Periapical radiolucency around maxillary permanent first bicuspid
O.    Carious lesion
P.    Periapical radiolucency around maxillary permanent lateral incisor
Q.    Palatal cusp of maxillary permanent second bicuspid
R.    Palatal cusp of maxillary permanent first bicuspid
S.    Resorbed root of maxillary permanent lateral incisor

Plate 15     MAXILLARY CUSPID REGION VIEW

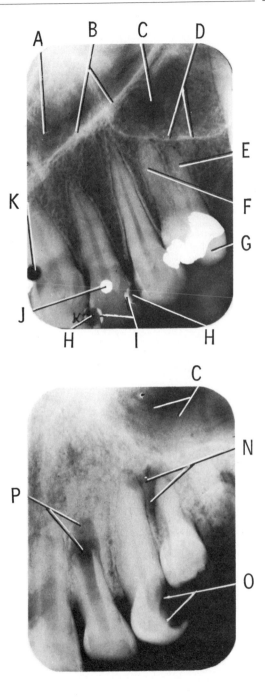

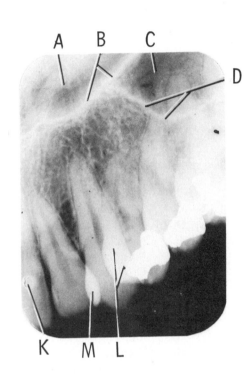

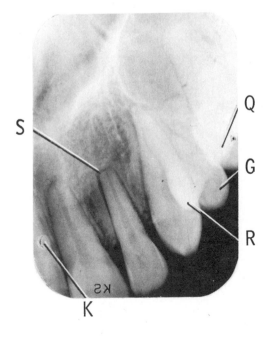

Plate 16     MAXILLARY INCISOR REGION VIEW _____

A.   Maxillary primary lateral incisor
B.   Unerupted maxillary permanent lateral incisor
C.   Developing root of erupting maxillary permanent central incisor
D.   Nasal fossa
E.   Nasal septum
F.   Median palatal suture
G.   Crowns of maxillary primary central incisors with resorbed roots
H.   Anterior nasal spine
I.   Mesiodens
J.   Opening made on lingual side of tooth for attempted endodontic treatment
K.   Erosion
L.   Endodontic filling material
M.   Silver alloy retrograde filling
N.   Resin restorations

Plate 16     MAXILLARY INCISOR REGION VIEW

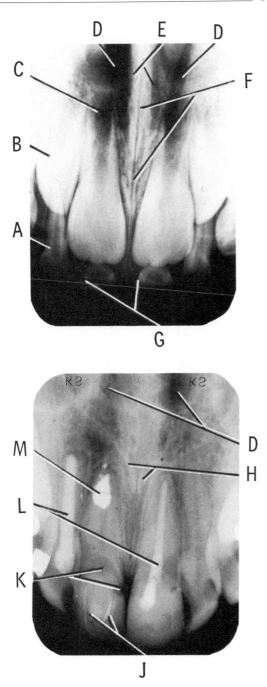

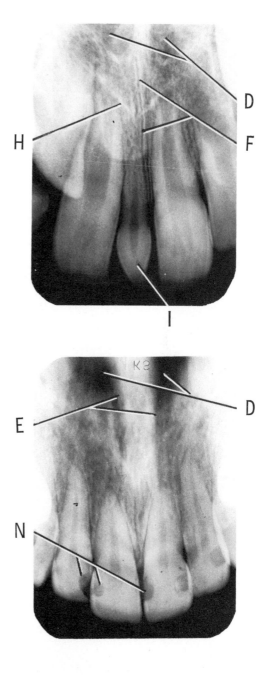

Plate 17    MAXILLARY INCISOR REGION VIEW _____

A.    Nasal fossa
B.    Nasal septum
C.    Anterior nasal spine
D.    Incisive foramen
E.    Lip line
F.    Lingual metal restoration
G.    Median palatal suture
H.    Film identification dot
I.    Anterior extent of maxillary sinus
J.    Carious lesion
K.    Gold pontic
L.    Gold crown restoration
M.    Surgical defect
N.    Soft tissue of nose

Plate 17     MAXILLARY INCISOR REGION VIEW

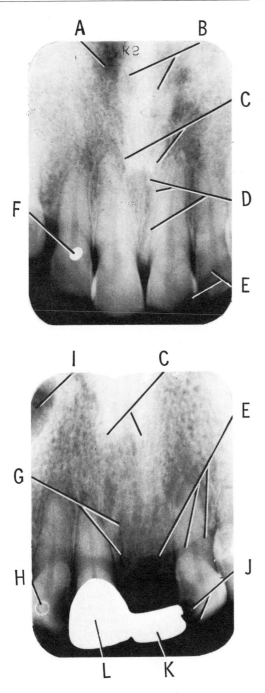

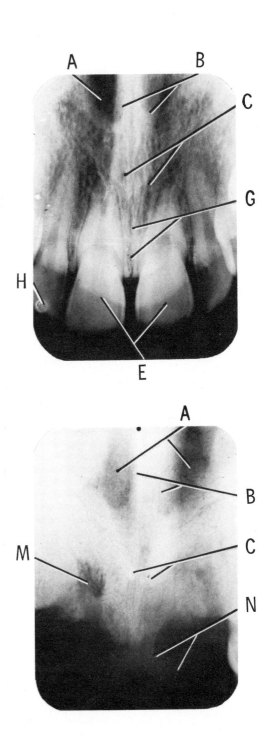

Plate 18    MAXILLARY INCISOR REGION VIEW _____

A.    Unerupted maxillary permanent cuspid
B.    Nasal septum
C.    Radiolucent line indicating cervical area and bone level
D.    Shadow of soft tissue of nose
E.    Gold pontics of anterior bridge
F.    Nasal fossa
G.    Supernumerary teeth
H.    Unerupted maxillary permanent lateral incisor
I.    Unerupted maxillary permanent central incisor
J.    Maxillary primary lateral incisor
K.    Maxillary primary central incisor

Plate 18    MAXILLARY INCISOR REGION VIEW

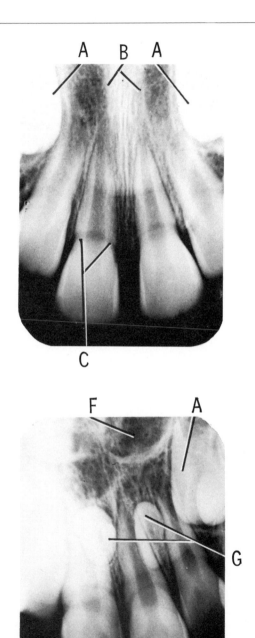

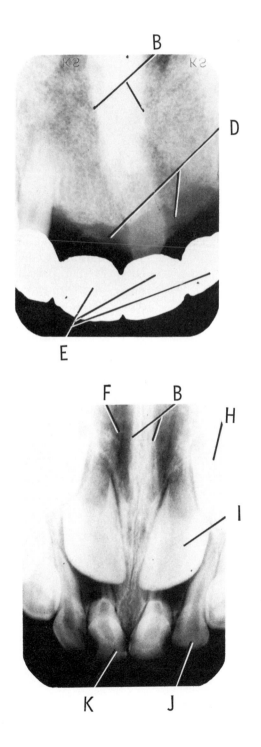

Plate 19    MAXILLARY INCISOR REGION VIEW _____

A.    Nasal fossa
B.    Anterior nasal spine
C.    Carious lesion
D.    Median palatal suture
E.    Incisive nerve foramen
F.    Periapical lesion
G.    Carious lesion involving pulp chamber
H.    Shadow of lip line
I.    Supernumerary tooth (mesiodens)
J.    Nasal septum
K.    Developing roots of maxillary permanent central incisors
L.    Crown remnants of maxillary primary lateral incisors

Plate 19    MAXILLARY INCISOR REGION VIEW

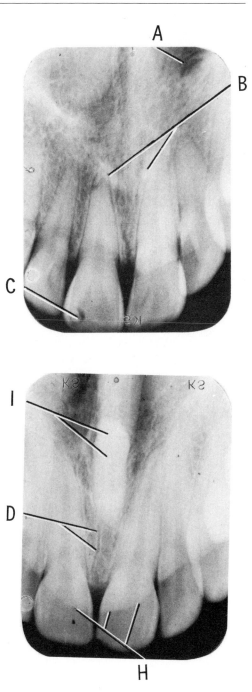

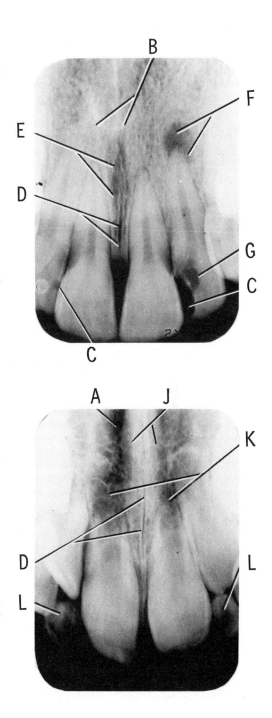

Plate 20     MAXILLARY INCISOR REGION VIEW

A.     Impacted maxillary permanent central incisor
B.     Nasal fossae
C.     Incisal attrition
D.     Resorbed root
E.     Gold post and core of endodontically treated maxillary permanent central incisors
F.     Reinforcing wire under resin restoration replacing fractured incisal edge
G.     Overlapping of maxillary permanent lateral and central incisors
H.     Crown fracture of maxillary permanent central incisor
I.     Shadow of lip line

Plate 20    MAXILLARY INCISOR REGION VIEW

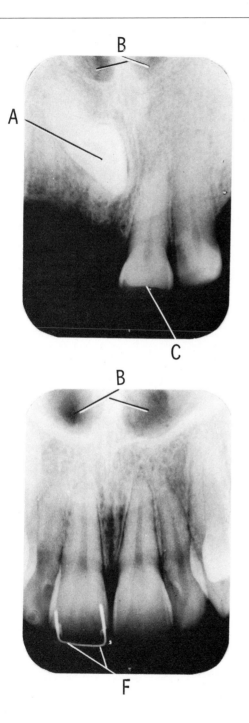

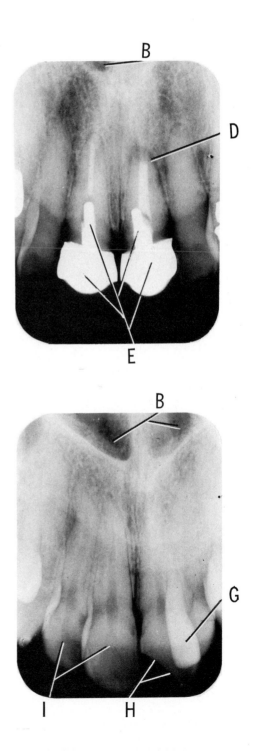

Plate 21     MAXILLARY INCISOR REGION VIEW

A.  Nasal conchae in nasal fossae
B.  Nasal fossae
C.  Anterior nasal spine
D.  Shadow of lip line
E.  Nasal septum
F.  Incisive nerve foramen
G.  Area of missing anterior restoration
H.  Carious lesion
I.  Median palatal suture
J.  Resorbed roots
K.  Resin restoration

Plate 21    MAXILLARY INCISOR REGION VIEW

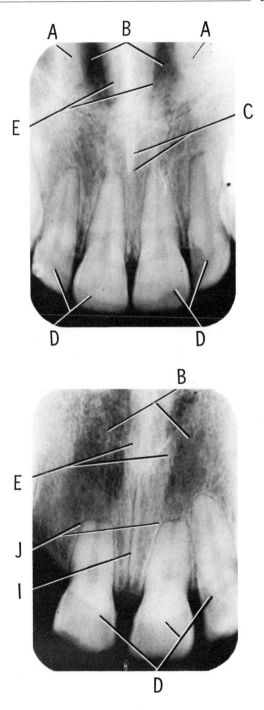

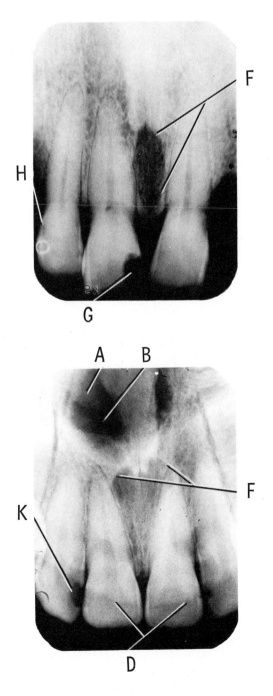

Plate 22    MAXILLARY INCISOR REGION VIEW _____

A.    Nasal fossa
B.    Nasal septum
C.    Film crease
D.    Impacted maxillary permanent cuspid
E.    Rubber material around metal film holder
F.    Metal film holder
G.    Soft tissue of nose
H.    Zinc oxide temporary restoration
I.    Anterior nasal spine
J.    Cement bases under resin restorations
K.    Carious lesion

Plate 22    MAXILLARY INCISOR REGION VIEW

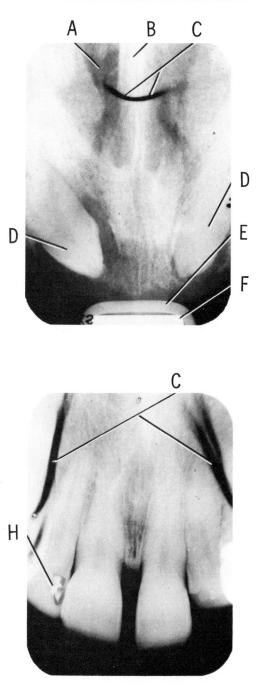

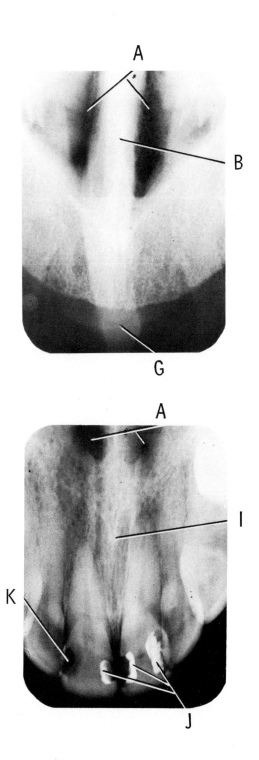

Plate 23     MANDIBULAR MOLAR REGION VIEW _____

A.     Mandibular canal
B.     Film identification dot
C.     External oblique ridge
D.     Cervical burnout (adumbration)
E.     Enamel pearl
F.     Internal oblique ridge
G.     Overhanging restoration
H.     Radiolucent normal bone area

Plate 23    MANDIBULAR MOLAR REGION VIEW

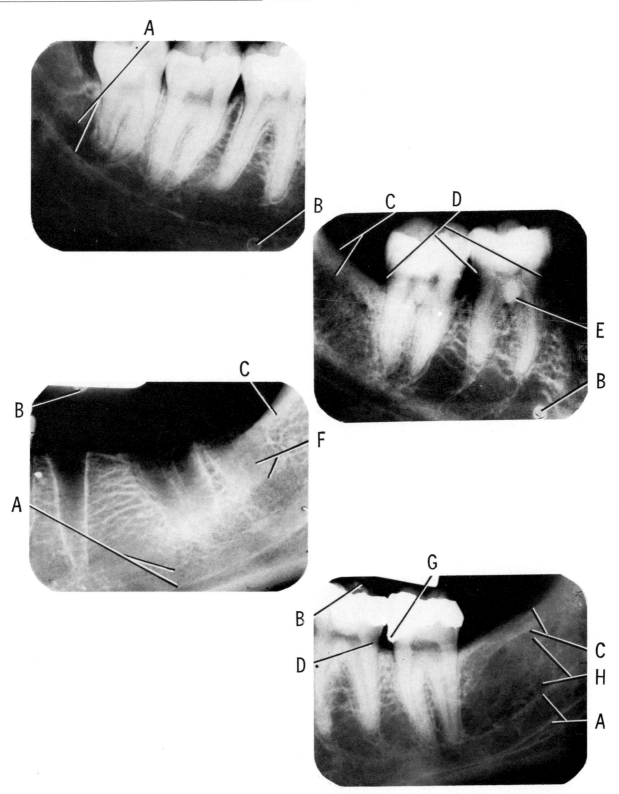

Plate 24     MANDIBULAR MOLAR REGION VIEW _____

A.     Recurrent caries
B.     Area of bone resorption
C.     Fused roots
D.     Dilacerated root
E.     Mandibular canal
F.     Healing extraction site

Plate 24     MANDIBULAR MOLAR REGION VIEW

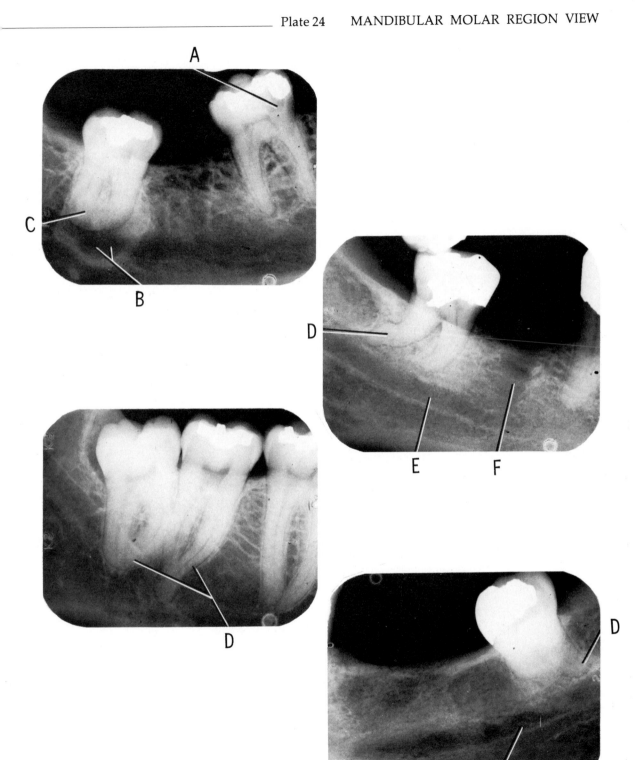

Plate 25     MANDIBULAR MOLAR REGION VIEW _____

**A.**     Pulp stone
**B.**     Retained root fragments
**C.**     Radiolucency indicating bone resorption
**D.**     Radiolucency indicating bone destruction due to periodontal disease
**E.**     Film identification dot
**F.**     Mandibular canal
**G.**     External oblique ridge
**H.**     Enamel pearl
**I.**     Cortical bone of inferior border of mandible
**J.**     Healing extraction site
**K.**     Tooth crown destruction due to caries
**L.**     Bone overlying developing permanent third molar
**M.**     Developing permanent third molar in follicle
**N.**     Early calcification of bifurcation of permanent third molar
**O.**     Periapical bone loss due to carious lesion
**P.**     Cervical burnout (adumbration)

Plate 25    MANDIBULAR MOLAR REGION VIEW

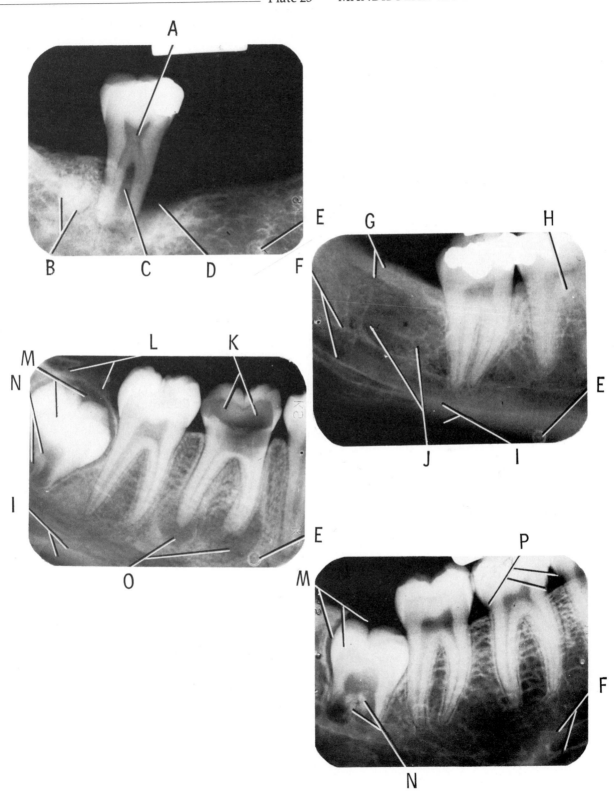

Plate 26    MANDIBULAR MOLAR REGION VIEW _____

A. Lamina dura of tooth follicle
B. Developing mandibular permanent third molar in follicle
C. Alveolar bone level
D. Developing roots of mandibular permanent second molar
E. Horizontal developing mandibular permanent third molar
F. Overhanging restoration
G. Horizontally impacted mandibular permanent third molar

Plate 26    MANDIBULAR MOLAR REGION VIEW

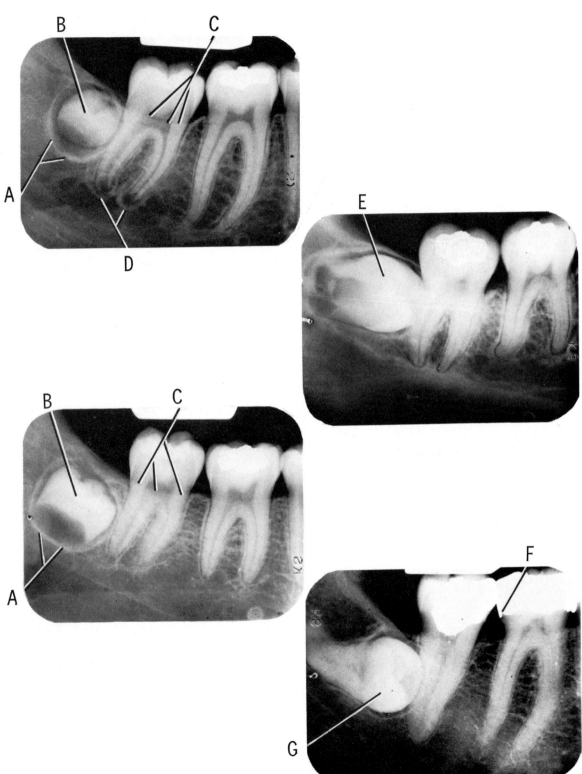

Plate 27    MANDIBULAR MOLAR REGION VIEW _____

A. External oblique ridge
B. Shadow of soft tissue
C. Carious lesion in permanent third molar
D. Portion of metal film holder
E. Carious lesion in permanent second molar
F. Normal bone trabeculation
G. Retained root tip in soft tissue
H. Distal surface of permanent second bicuspid
I. Mandibular canal
J. Film identification dot
K. Radiolucent area indicating bone loss due to cariously infected tooth
L. Lamina dura at alveolar bone crest
M. Bone located over unerupted permanent third molar
N. Unerupted developing permanent third molar located in developing tooth follicle
O. Incompletely developed apices
P. Periodontal ligament space (radiolucent line)
Q. Cortical bone of inferior border of mandible
R. Silver restoration
S. Zinc phosphate cement base
T. Gold full crown
U. Distal root canal
V. Interradicular bone
W. Follicle of developing tooth
X. Mesially impacted permanent third molar
Y. Overlapping contacts of permanent molars
Z. Apex of mesial root of permanent first molar

Plate 27    MANDIBULAR MOLAR REGION VIEW

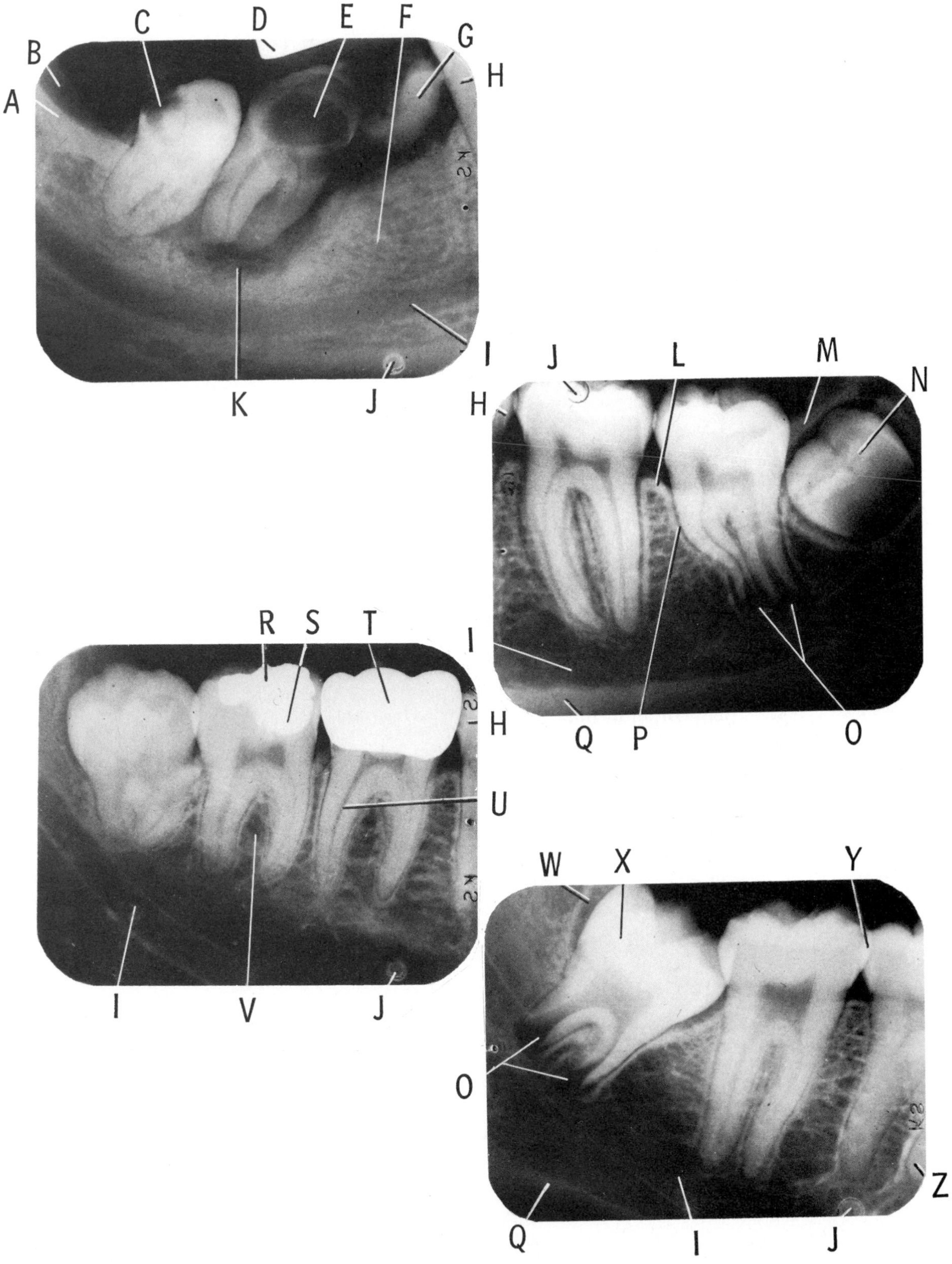

Plate 28     MANDIBULAR MOLAR REGION VIEW _____

A.     Distally impacted mandibular permanent third molar
B.     Medullary bone resorbed indicating possible cyst formation
C.     Mandibular canal
D.     Cortical bone of inferior border of mandible
E.     Internal oblique ridge
F.     Developing crown of mandibular permanent third molar
G.     Portion of metal film holder
H.     Film identification dot
I.     Rubber material surrounding film holder
J.     Resorbed roots of mandibular permanent first molar
K.     Bent corner of film

Plate 28    MANDIBULAR MOLAR REGION VIEW

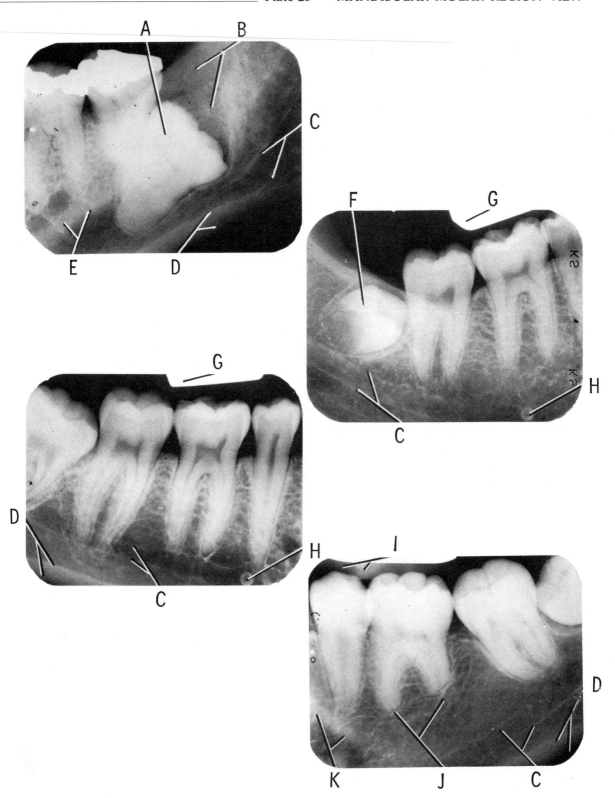

Plate 29    MANDIBULAR  BICUSPID  REGION  VIEW _____

A.    Zinc phosphate cement base
B.    Silver restoration
C.    Cast gold restoration
D.    Portion of metal film holder
E.    Rubber material surrounding film holder
F.    Cervical burnout (adumbration)
G.    Bent corner of film
H.    Mental foramen
I.    Mandibular canal
J.    Alveolar bone ridge
K.    External oblique ridge
L.    Internal oblique ridge
M.    Submandibular fossa
N.    Cast gold crown bridge abutment
O.    Cast gold bridge pontics
P.    Healed extraction sites

Plate 29    MANDIBULAR BICUSPID REGION VIEW

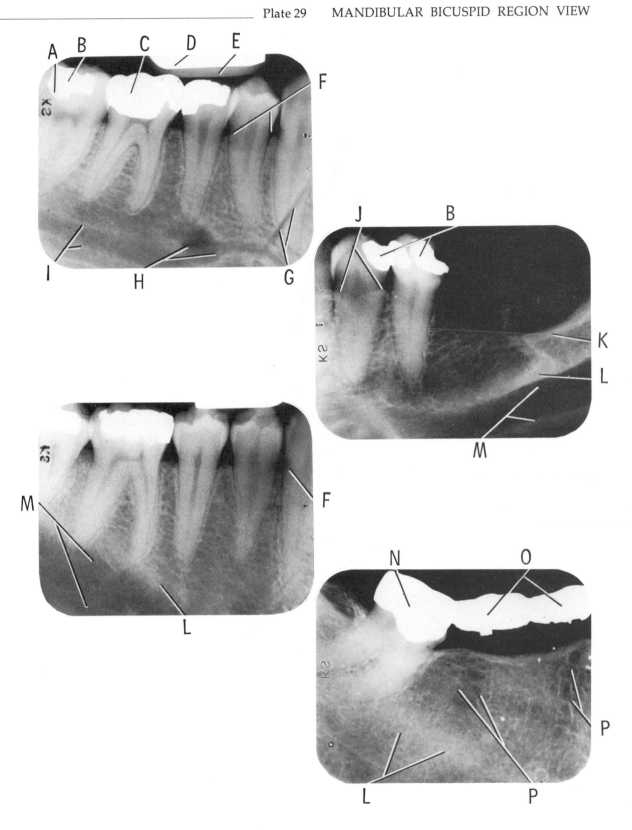

Plate 30     MANDIBULAR BICUSPID REGION VIEW _____

A.     Mandibular permanent cuspid
B.     Film identification dot
C.     Crown of resorbed mandibular primary first molar
D.     Mandibular primary second molar
E.     Erupting mandibular permanent second molar
F.     Incompletely developed roots of mandibular permanent first molar
G.     Developing crown of mandibular permanent second bicuspid
H.     Developing mandibular permanent first bicuspid
I.     Incompletely developed root of mandibular permanent first bicuspid
J.     Lingual cusp of mandibular permanent first bicuspid
K.     Portion of metal film holder
L.     Supernumerary mandibular bicuspid
M.     Submandibular fossa
N.     Dilacerated mesial root of mandibular permanent first molar
O.     Mental foramen
P.     Buccal cusps of mandibular permanent first molar
Q.     Unerupted mandibular permanent cuspid
R.     Lingual cusps of mandibular permanent first molar
S.     Follicle of developing permanent second molar

Plate 30    MANDIBULAR BICUSPID REGION VIEW

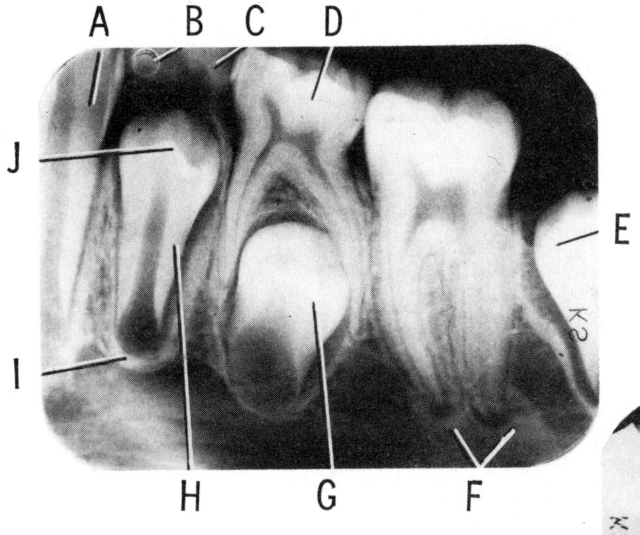

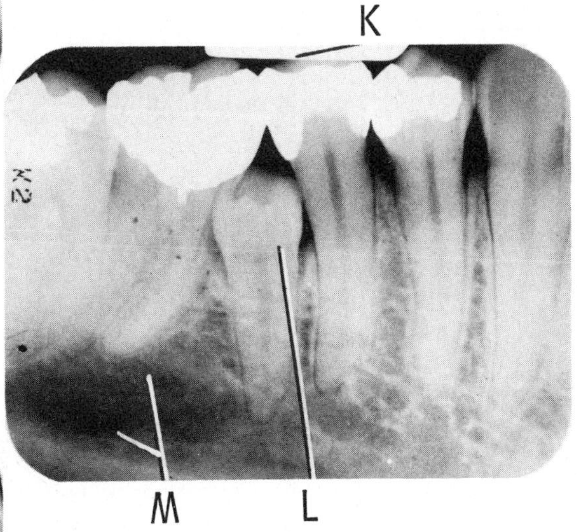

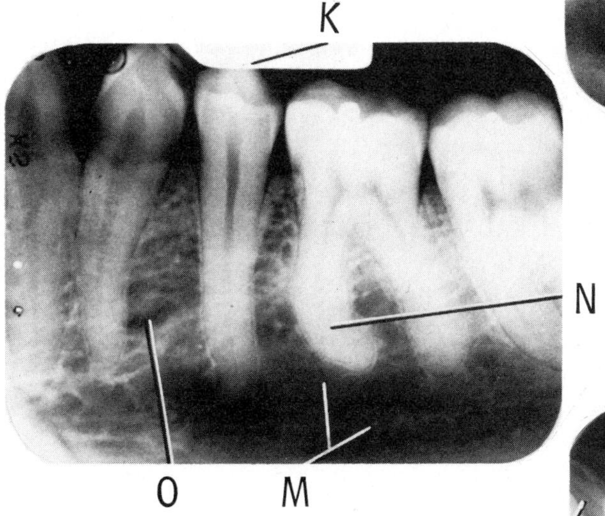

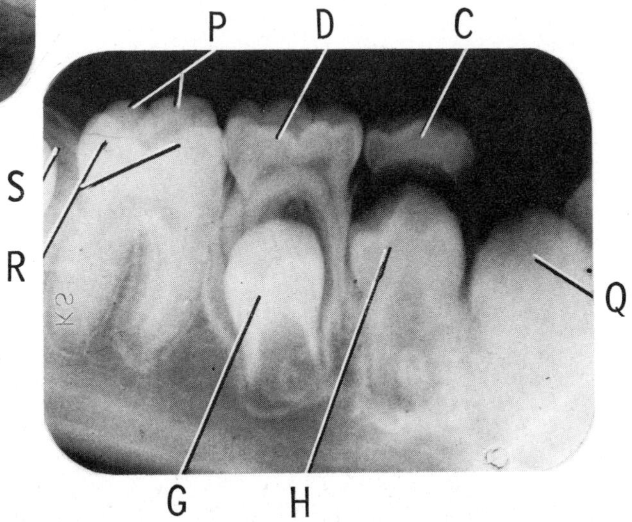

Plate 31    MANDIBULAR BICUSPID REGION VIEW _____

A.    Torn film emulsion
B.    Buccal cusp of mandibular permanent first bicuspid
C.    Lingual cusp of mandibular permanent first bicuspid
D.    Portion of metal film holder
E.    Metal restorations
F.    Submandibular fossa
G.    Internal oblique ridge
H.    Mandibular canal
I.    Mental foramen
J.    Sclerotic bone
K.    Film identification dot
L.    Shadow of portion of wooden film holder
M.    Resorbed edentulous ridge
N.    Bent corner of film
O.    Cortical bone of inferior border of mandible
P.    Bifid root of mandibular permanent second bicuspid
Q.    Hypercementosed distal root—mandibular permanent first molar
R.    Mandibular primary cuspid
S.    Pulpally treated mandibular primary first molar
T.    Chrome steel crown
U.    Pulpally treated mandibular primary second molar
V.    Buccal cusps of mandibular first molar
W.    Partial view of unerupted mandibular permanent second molar
X.    Developing mandibular second bicuspid
Y.    Developing mandibular permanent first bicuspid
Z.    Developing mandibular permanent cuspid

Plate 31    MANDIBULAR BICUSPID REGION VIEW

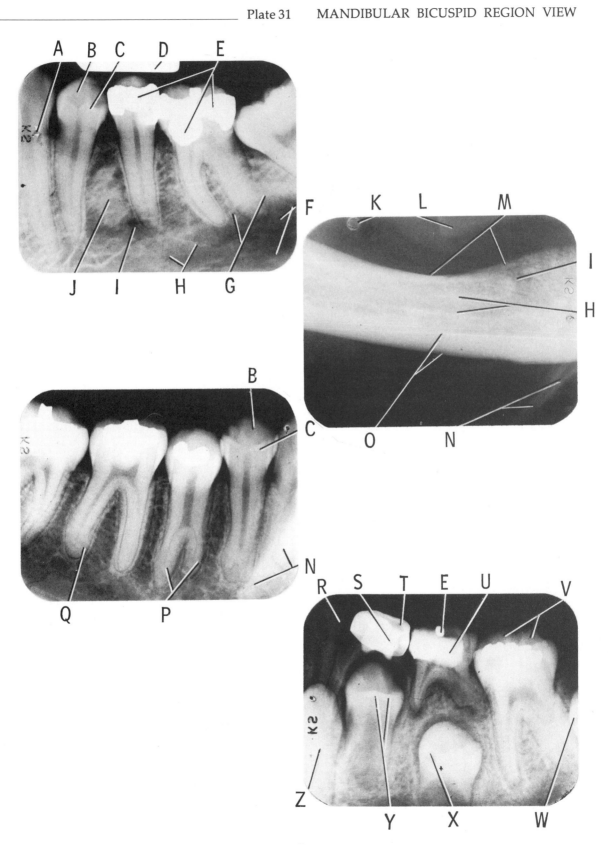

Plate 32    MANDIBULAR BICUSPID REGION VIEW _____

**A.**    Supernumerary teeth
**B.**    Nutrient foramen

Plate 32    MANDIBULAR BICUSPID REGION VIEW

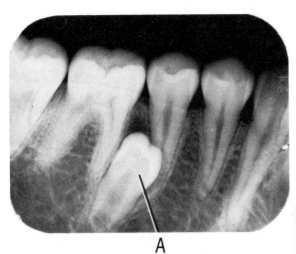

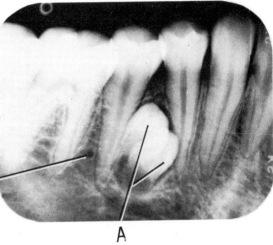

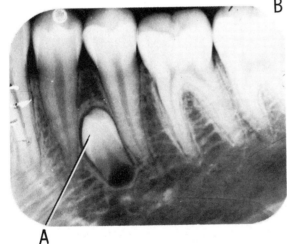

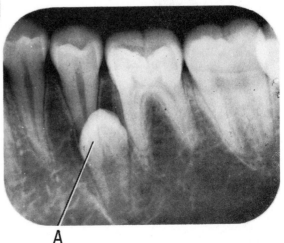

Plate 33    MANDIBULAR BICUSPID–MOLAR REGION VIEW _____

A.   Pulp canal recession due to indirect pulp capping procedure
B.   Cervical burnout (adumbration)
C.   Mental foramen
D.   Film crease
E.   Sclerotic bone (osteosclerosis)
F.   Mandibular canal
G.   Portion of impacted mandibular permanent third molar
H.   Carious lesions
I.   Condensing osteitis
J.   Radiolucency indicating pulpal pathology, probably due to operative pulp damage
K.   Periodontal interradicular radiolucency indicating bone resorption and pathology
L.   Radiolucency around crown of erupting mandibular permanent second bicuspid
M.   Developing root of mandibular permanent second bicuspid
N.   Submandibular fossa

Plate 33 MANDIBULAR BICUSPID–MOLAR REGION VIEW

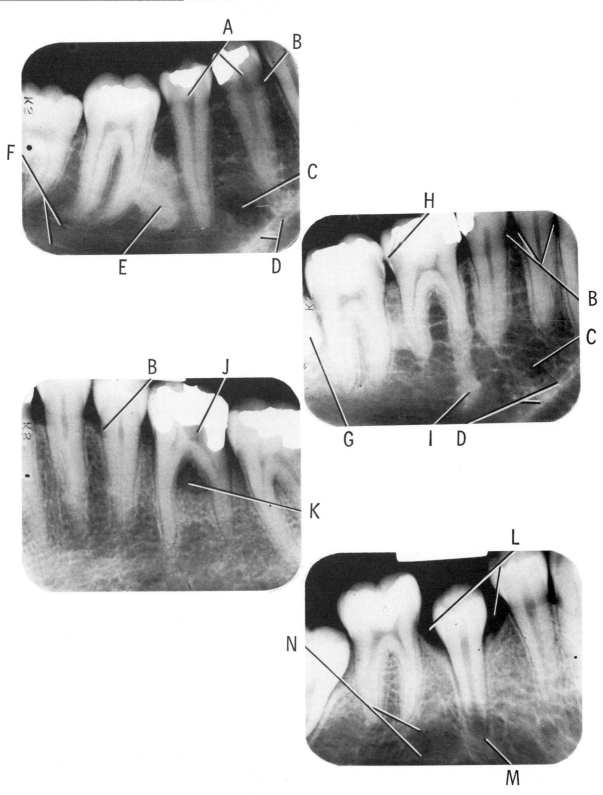

Plate 34    MANDIBULAR BICUSPID–MOLAR REGION VIEW _____

A.    Internal oblique ridge
B.    External oblique ridge
C.    Film identification dot
D.    Mandibular canal
E.    Dilacerated roots
F.    Portion of metal film holder
G.    Remnant of primary second molar
H.    Area of resorbed bone over erupting permanent second molar
I.    Follicle of developing permanent second bicuspid
J.    Caries
K.    Submandibular fossa

Plate 34     MANDIBULAR BICUSPID–MOLAR REGION VIEW

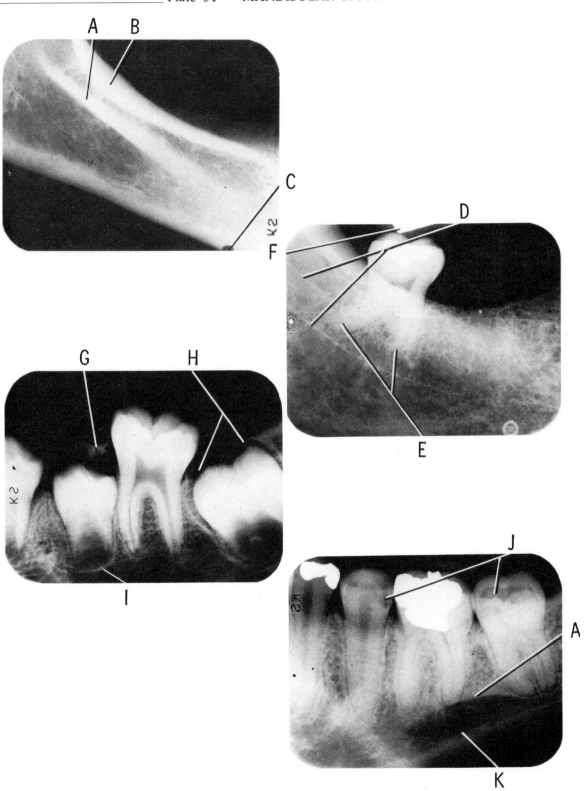

Plate 35    MANDIBULAR BICUSPID–MOLAR REGION VIEW _____

A.    Submandibular fossa
B.    Ankylosed mandibular primary second molar with no developing permanent second bicuspid
C.    Alveolar bone level
D.    Film identification dot
E.    Lingual cusp of mandibular permanent first bicuspid
F.    Buccal cusp of mandibular permanent first bicuspid
G.    Impacted mandibular permanent second bicuspid
H.    Chrome steel band and loop space maintainer
I.    Metal portion of film holder
J.    Crown of developing mandibular permanent second bicuspid
K.    Crown of developing mandibular permanent first bicuspid
L.    Retained remnant of primary molar root

Plate 35    MANDIBULAR BICUSPID–MOLAR REGION VIEW

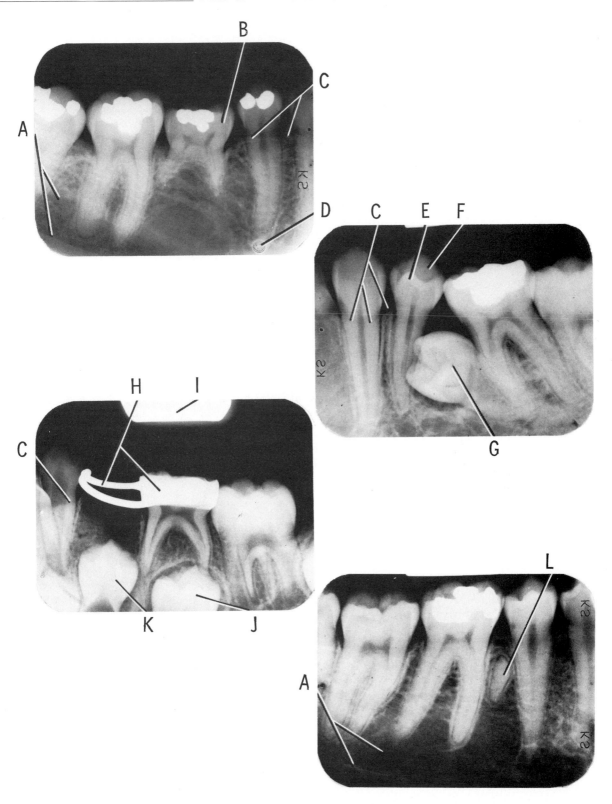

Plate 36     MANDIBULAR BICUSPID–MOLAR REGION VIEW _____

**A.** Film crease
**B.** Mental foramen
**C.** Cortical bone of inferior border of mandible
**D.** Overhanging metal restorations
**E.** Mandibular canal
**F.** Extraction site of mandibular molar
**G.** Extraction site of mandibular bicuspid
**H.** Lamina dura
**I.** Retained root tip in soft tissue
**J.** Large carious lesion

Plate 36     MANDIBULAR BICUSPID–MOLAR REGION VIEW

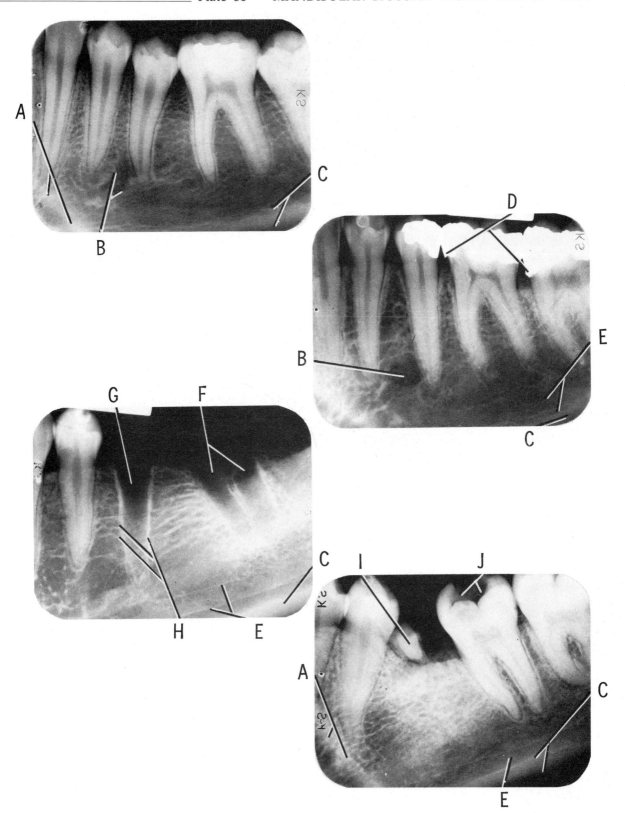

Plate 37    MANDIBULAR CUSPID REGION VIEW _____

A.    Enamel hypoplasia
B.    Internal oblique ridge
C.    Submandibular fossa
D.    Cortical plate of inferior border of mandible
E.    Mandibular primary lateral incisor
F.    Mandibular primary cuspid
G.    Mandibular primary first molar
H.    Mandibular primary second molar
I.    Mandibular permanent first bicuspid
J.    Mandibular permanent second bicuspid
K.    Mandibular permanent cuspid
L.    Mandibular permanent lateral incisor

Plate 37    MANDIBULAR CUSPID REGION VIEW

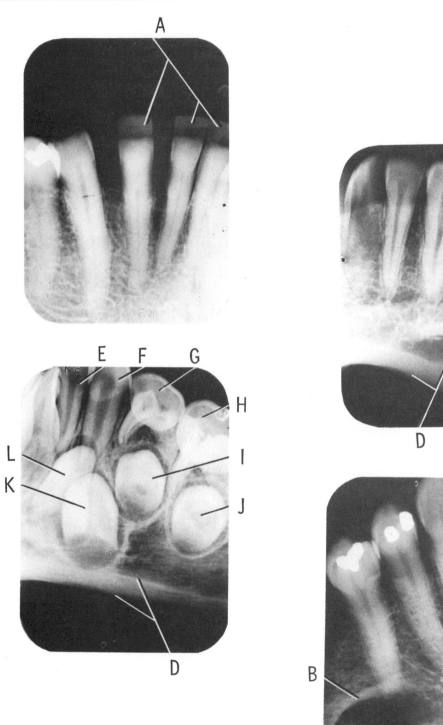
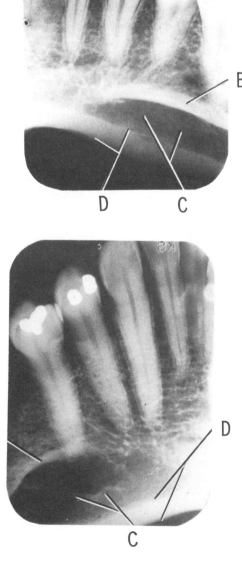

Plate 38     MANDIBULAR CUSPID REGION VIEW _____

A.    Lip line
B.    Area of bone loss
C.    Alveolar bone ridge line
D.    Cervical abrasion
E.    Sclerotic bone
F.    Calculus
G.    Metal film holder
H.    Genial tubercle
I.    Lingual foramen
J.    Impacted mandibular permanent cuspid

Plate 38    MANDIBULAR CUSPID REGION VIEW

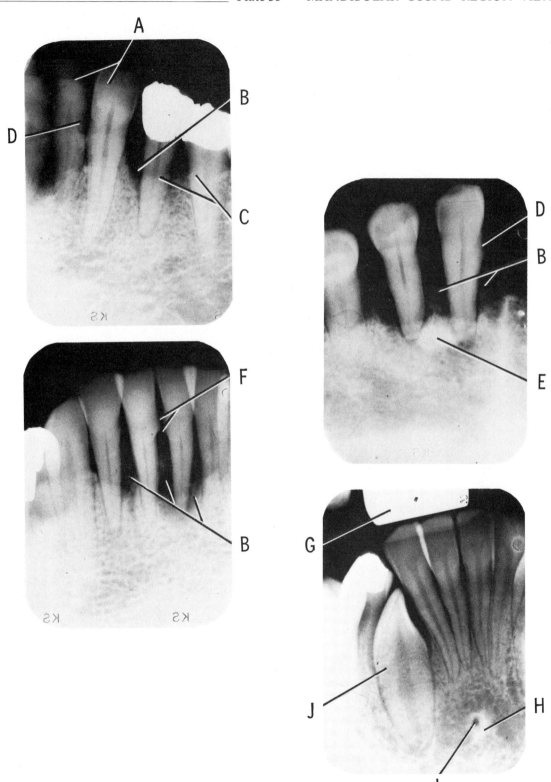

Plate 39     MANDIBULAR CUSPID REGION VIEW _____

A.    Cervical burnout (adumbration)
B.    Shadow of alveolar bone level
C.    Calculus
D.    Area of bone resorption
E.    Developing mandibular permanent cuspid
F.    Exfoliating mandibular primary molar
G.    Developing root of mandibular permanent cuspid
H.    Cortical bone of inferior border of mandible
I.    Shadow of wooden film holder
J.    Superimposition of mandibular permanent first bicuspid over permanent cuspid

Plate 39    MANDIBULAR CUSPID REGION VIEW

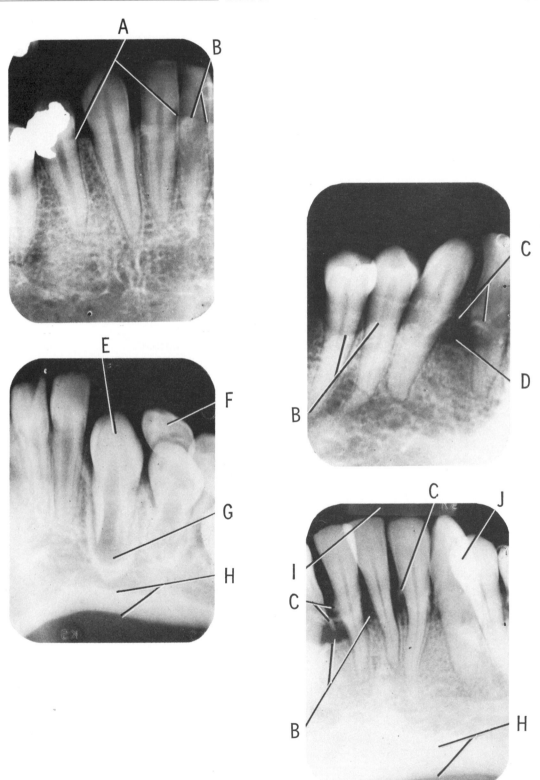

Plate 40    MANDIBULAR  CUSPID  REGION  VIEW _____

A.    Unerupted mandibular permanent cuspid in follicle
B.    Mandibular primary first molar
C.    Mandibular primary cuspid — root resorbed
D.    Cortical bone of inferior border of mandible
E.    Recurrent caries
F.    Periapical radiolucency due to large carious lesions
G.    Alveolar bone level
H.    Normal trabecular bone pattern
I.    Occlusal and incisal abrasion
J.    Fixer chemical stain

Plate 40   MANDIBULAR CUSPID REGION VIEW

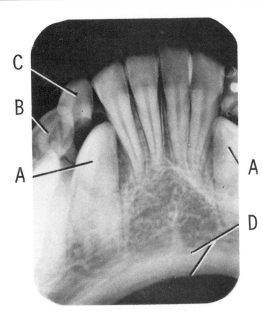

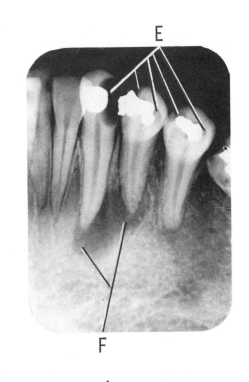

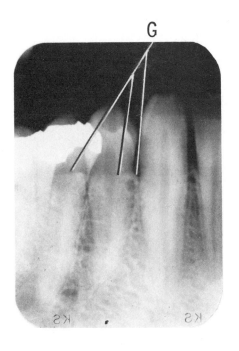

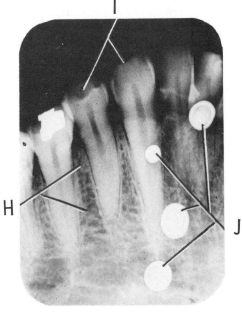

Plate 41     MANDIBULAR INCISOR REGION VIEW _____

A.   Fractured enamel
B.   Overlapped contacts
C.   Abrasion
D.   Level of alveolar bone
E.   Lingual foramen
F.   Lip line
G.   Genial tubercle
H.   Film crease
I.   Cortical bone—inferior border of mandible
J.   Narrow pulp canal (due to attrition)
K.   Sclerosed pulp chamber (due to attrition)
L.   Attrition
M.   Mamelons
N.   Film identification dot
O.   Radiolucency of follicle around unerupted permanent cuspid

Plate 41     MANDIBULAR INCISOR REGION VIEW

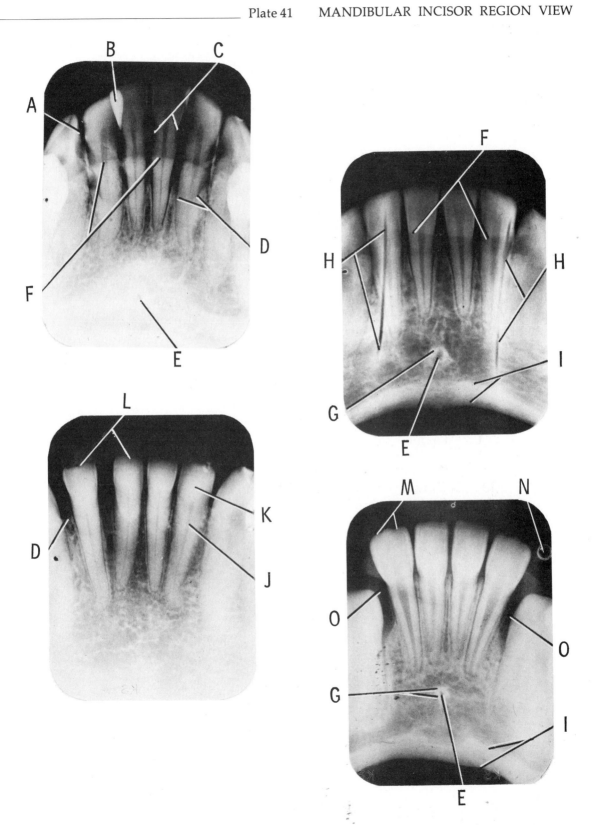

Plate 42    MANDIBULAR INCISOR REGION VIEW

A.    Radiolucent resin restorations
B.    Normal thin bone
C.    Genial tubercle
D.    Incisal abrasion
E.    Radiopaque calculus bridge
F.    Alveolar ridge bone line
G.    Nutrient foramen
H.    Nutrient canals
I.    Lip line
J.    Mental ridge
K.    Unerupted mandibular permanent cuspid
L.    Cortical bone of inferior border of mandible
M.    Gold crown restoration of mandibular permanent cuspid

Plate 42   MANDIBULAR INCISOR REGION VIEW

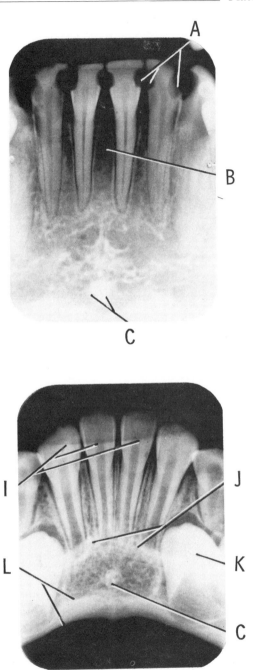

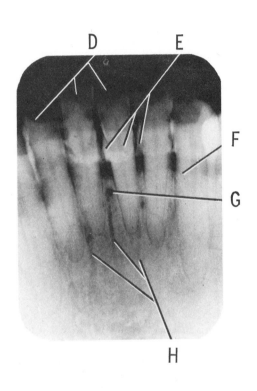

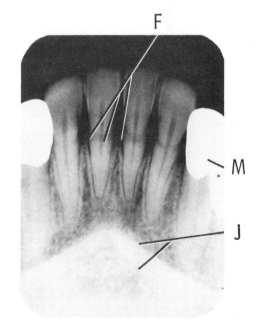

Plate 43     MANDIBULAR INCISOR REGION VIEW _____

A.    Permanent lateral incisor
B.    Permanent central incisor
C.    Overlapping contacts
D.    Permanent cuspid
E.    Genial tubercle
F.    Lingual foramen
G.    Inferior cortical plate of border of mandible
H.    Enamel
I.    Shadow of lip
J.    Calculus
K.    Alveolar bone ridge
L.    Metal film holder
M.    Rubber material surrounding film holder
N.    Film identification dot
O.    Line of fracture
P.    Metal wire used to repair fracture
Q.    Developing permanent lateral incisors in follicles
R.    Permanent central incisors with incompletely developed roots
S.    Primary lateral incisor
T.    Primary cuspid

Plate 43    MANDIBULAR INCISOR REGION VIEW

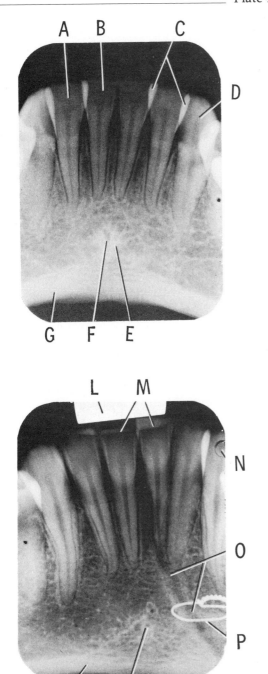

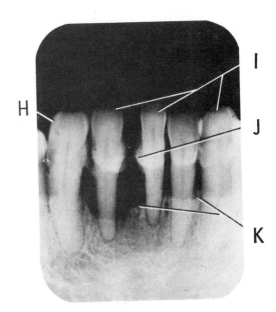

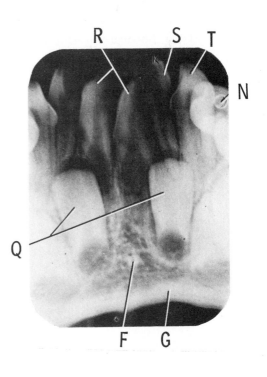

Plate 44    BITEWING VIEW OF BICUSPID–MOLAR REGION _____

A.    External oblique ridge
B.    Overcontoured gold crown restoration
C.    Healed extraction site
D.    Fractured area of crown
E.    Maxillary full denture prosthetic teeth
F.    Metal pin on lingual side of prosthetic cuspid tooth
G.    Radiolucent space between gold restoration and tooth preparation
H.    Endodontic filling material
I.    Portion of mandibular permanent molar
J.    Pulp stones
K.    Cervical burnout (adumbration)
L.    Maxillary tuberosity

Plate 44    BITEWING VIEW OF BICUSPID–MOLAR REGION

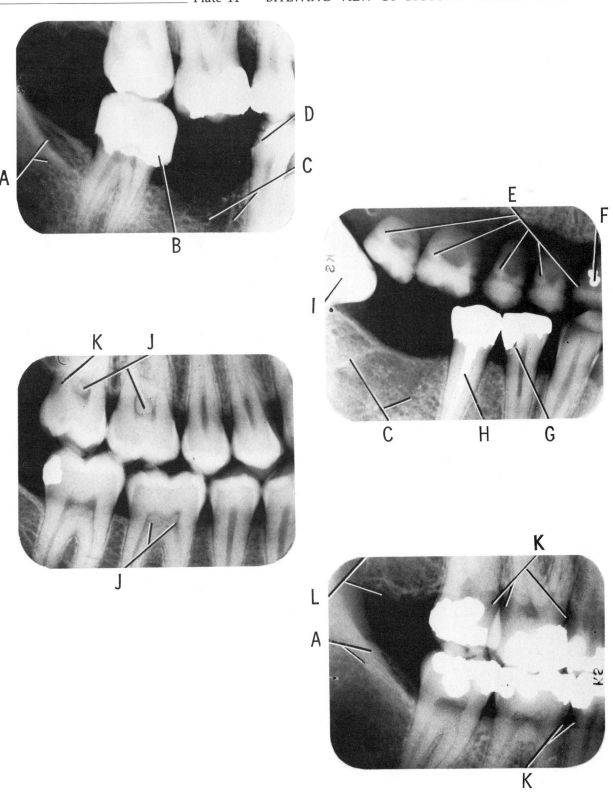

Plate 45     BITEWING VIEW OF BICUSPID–MOLAR REGION _____

A.     Endodontic restoration material
B.     Overhanging restoration
C.     Gold crown restoration
D.     Bone level
E.     Metal reinforcing pins under gold crown restoration are not in pulp
       chamber
F.     Floor of the maxillary sinus
G.     External oblique ridge of mandible
H.     Cervical burnout (adumbration)
I.     Film identification dot
J.     Portion of unerupted mandibular permanent third molar

Plate 45    BITEWING VIEW OF BICUSPID–MOLAR REGION

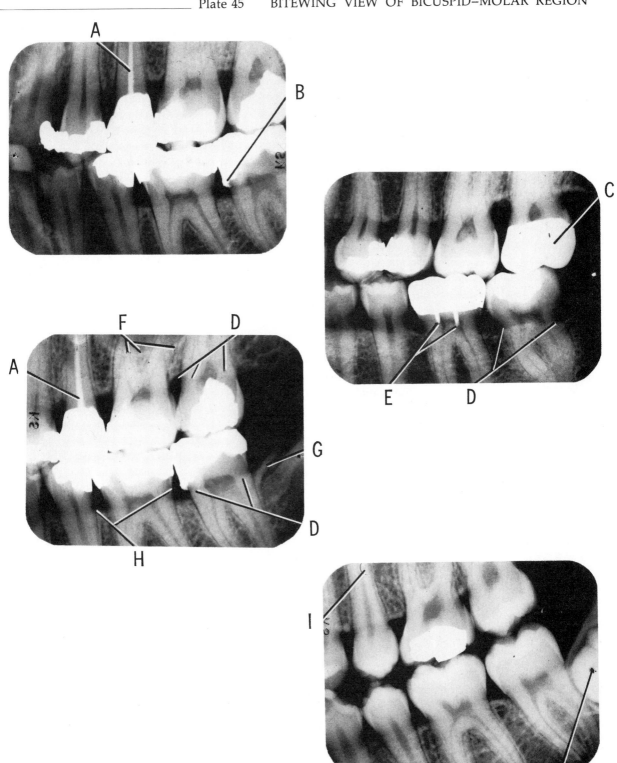

Plate 46    BITEWING VIEW OF BICUSPID–MOLAR REGION _____

A.    Pulp stone
B.    Cement base under silver alloy restoration
C.    Silver alloy restoration in buccal pit
D.    Root canal
E.    Enamel
F.    Pulp chamber
G.    Carious lesion

Plate 46     BITEWING VIEW OF BICUSPID–MOLAR REGION

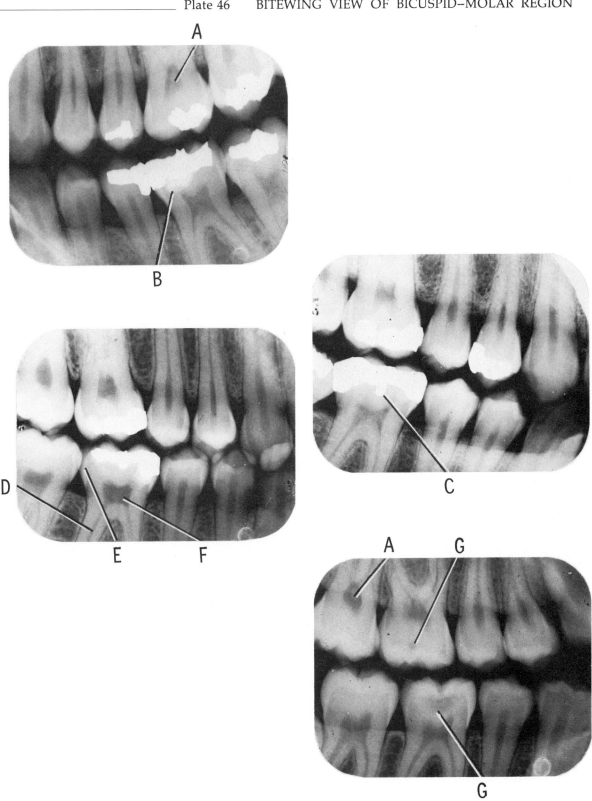

Plate 47    BITEWING VIEW OF BICUSPID–MOLAR REGION

A.    Poorly contoured silver alloy restoration
B.    Carious lesion
C.    Recurrent carious lesion
D.    Pulp stone
E.    Cement base under silver alloy restoration
F.    Secondary dentin
G.    Level of alveolar bone
H.    Erupting maxillary permanent second bicuspid
I.    Crown remnant of maxillary primary second molar

Plate 47    BITEWING VIEW OF BICUSPID–MOLAR REGION

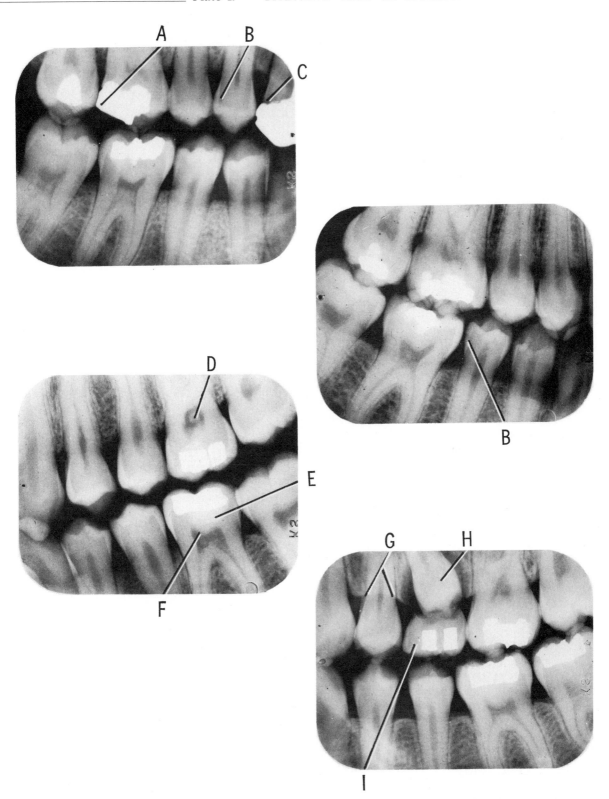

Plate 48     MAXILLARY ANTERIOR OCCLUSAL VIEW _____

A.   Nasal septum
B.   Nasal fossa
C.   Anterior nasal spine
D.   Nasal concha
E.   Impacted permanent central incisor
F.   Cone cut
G.   Fractured crown, permanent lateral incisor
H.   Periapical radiolucency
I.   Incisive foramen
J.   Median palatal suture
K.   Maxillary sinus
L.   Zygomatic process of maxilla

Plate 48     MAXILLARY ANTERIOR OCCLUSAL VIEW

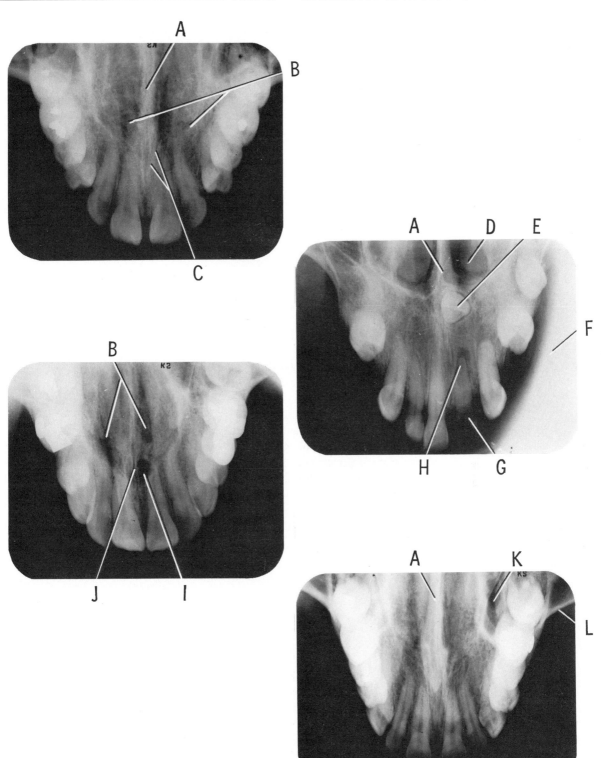

Plate 49     MAXILLARY ANTERIOR OCCLUSAL VIEW _____

A.  Nasal fossa
B.  Nasal septum
C.  Median palatal suture
D.  Maxillary sinus
E.  Anterior nasal spine
F.  Root canal filling
G.  Jacket crown preparation
H.  Superior foramina of incisive canal
I.  Cone cut
J.  Gold crown restorations
K.  Zygomatic process of maxilla
L.  Lateral border of nasal fossa
M.  Cartilaginous septum of nose
N.  Nasolacrimal duct
O.  Porcelain denture teeth with metal pins
P.  Retained root
Q.  Retained impacted tooth

Plate 49      MAXILLARY ANTERIOR OCCLUSAL VIEW

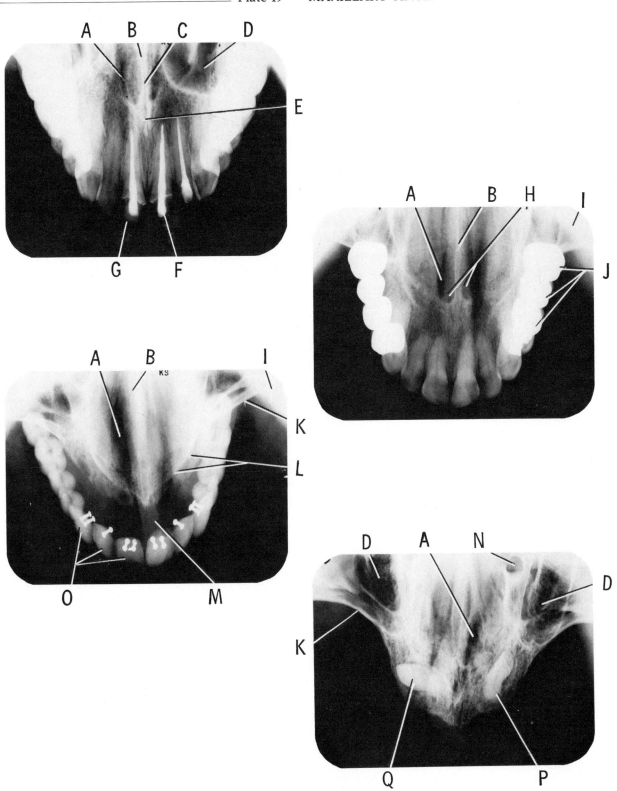

Plate 50     MANDIBULAR ANTERIOR OCCLUSAL VIEW _____

**A.**   Mental ridge
**B.**   Genial tubercle
**C.**   External oblique ridge
**D.**   Shadow of tongue
**E.**   Cone cut

Plate 50    MANDIBULAR ANTERIOR OCCLUSAL VIEW

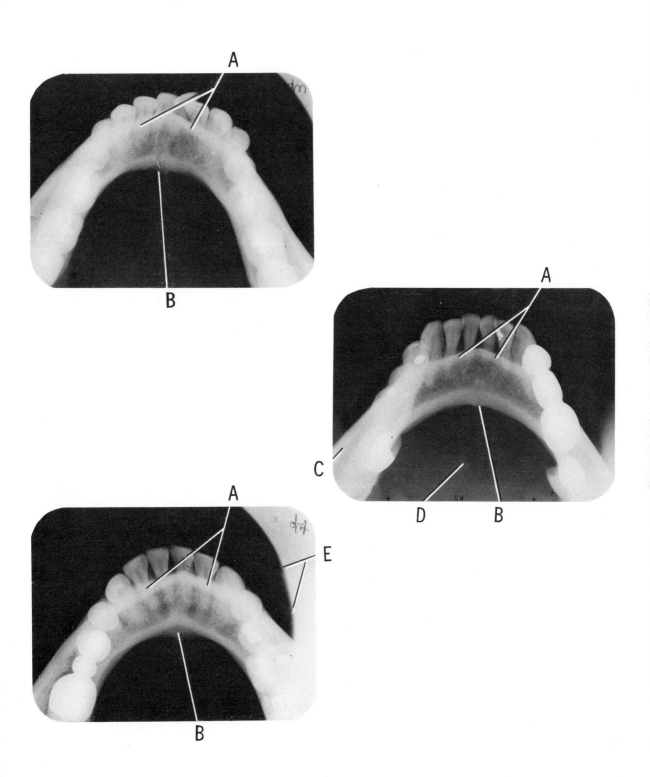

# section two

# EXTRAORAL RADIOGRAPHS OF THE HUMAN SKULL

Plate 51     LATERAL OBLIQUE JAW VIEW _____

A.     Shadow of spinal vertebrae
B.     Zygomatic arch
C.     Coronoid process of mandible
D.     Shadow of the tongue
E.     Inferior border of opposite side of mandible
F.     Mental foramen
G.     Mandibular canal
H.     Hyoid bone
I.     Maxillary arch
J.     Wire used to repair earlier fracture
K.     Posterior wall of pharynx
L.     Mandibular condyle

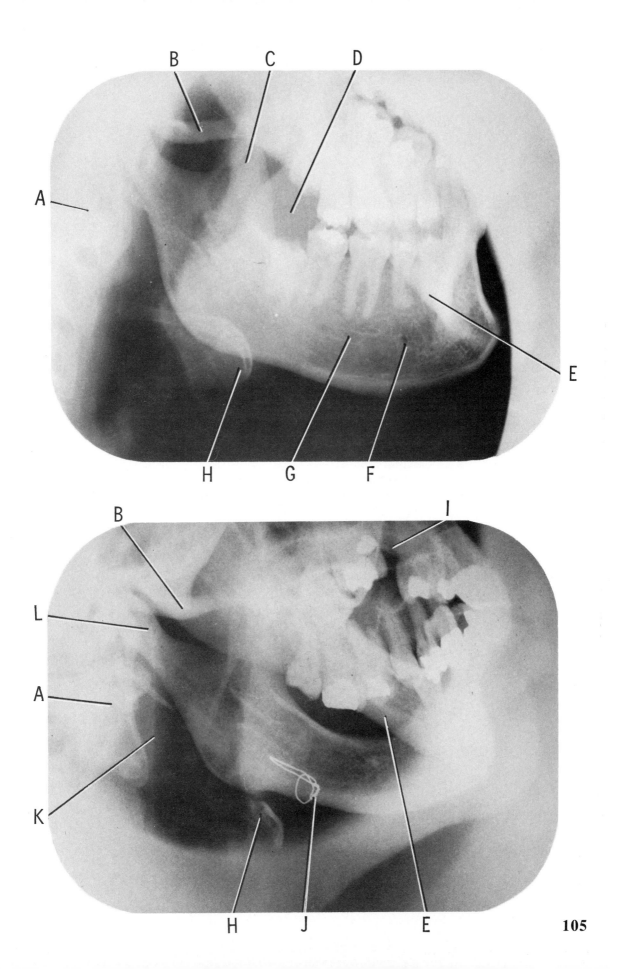

Plate 52     LATERAL OBLIQUE JAW VIEW _____

A.     Maxillary sinus
B.     Inferior border of opposite side of mandible
C.     Mental foramen
D.     Hyoid bone
E.     Cortical bone of inferior border of mandible
F.     Shadow of spinal vertebrae
G.     External oblique ridge
H.     Mandibular canal
I.     Mandibular foramen
J.     Sigmoid notch
K.     Coronoid process
L.     Zygomatic arch

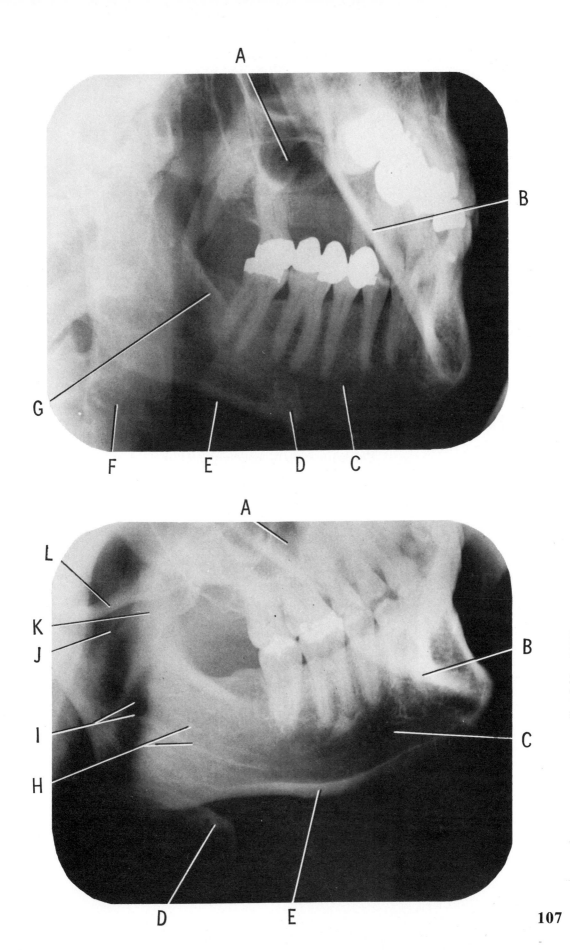

Plate 53    LATERAL OBLIQUE JAW VIEW _____

 

**A.**    Oropharynx
**B.**    Shadow of tongue
**C.**    Porcelain teeth of maxillary denture
**D.**    Mental foramen
**E.**    Mandibular canal
**F.**    Mandibular condyle
**G.**    Articular eminence
**H.**    Zygomatic arch
**I.**    Coronoid process of mandible
**J.**    Facial artery notch
**K.**    Styloid process

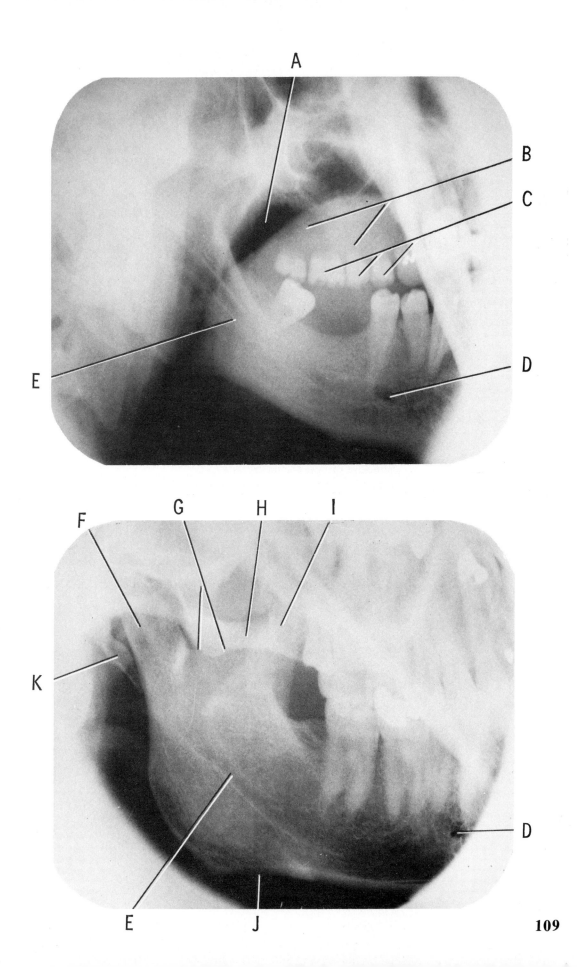

Plate 54     LATERAL OBLIQUE JAW VIEW _____

A.     Zygomatic arch
B.     Shadow of soft tissue of face
C.     Inferior border of opposite side of mandible
D.     Mental foramen
E.     Mandibular canal
F.     External oblique ridge
G.     Wall of pharynx
H.     Styloid process

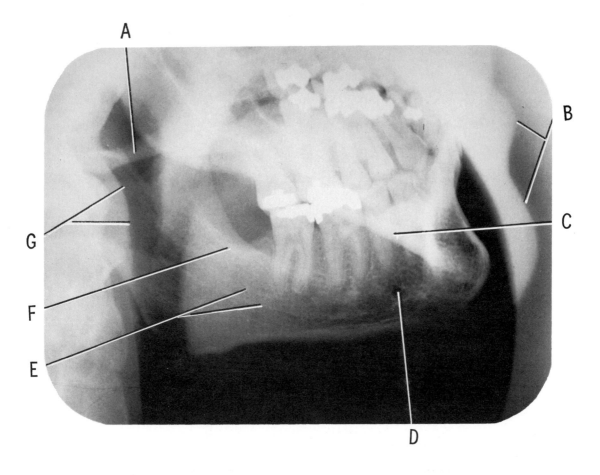

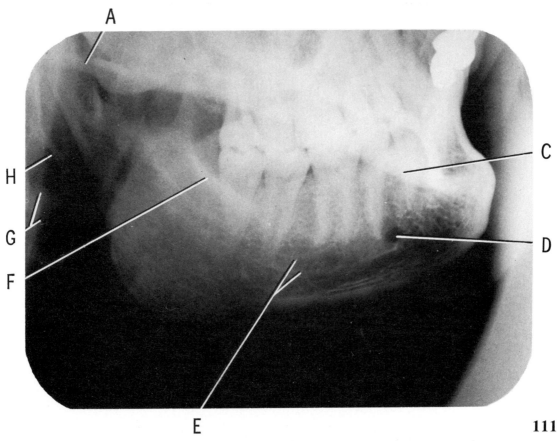

Plate 55    PANORAMIC VIEW _____

A.  Maxillary tuberosity
B.  Shadow of hard palate
C.  Zygoma
D.  Maxillary sinus
E.  Coronoid process of mandible
F.  Articular eminence
G.  Glenoid fossa
H.  Mandibular condyle
I.  Styloid process
J.  Mandibular canal
K.  External oblique ridge
L.  Metal bite-block
M.  Shadow of tongue
N.  Space between tongue and soft palate
O.  Shadow of soft palate

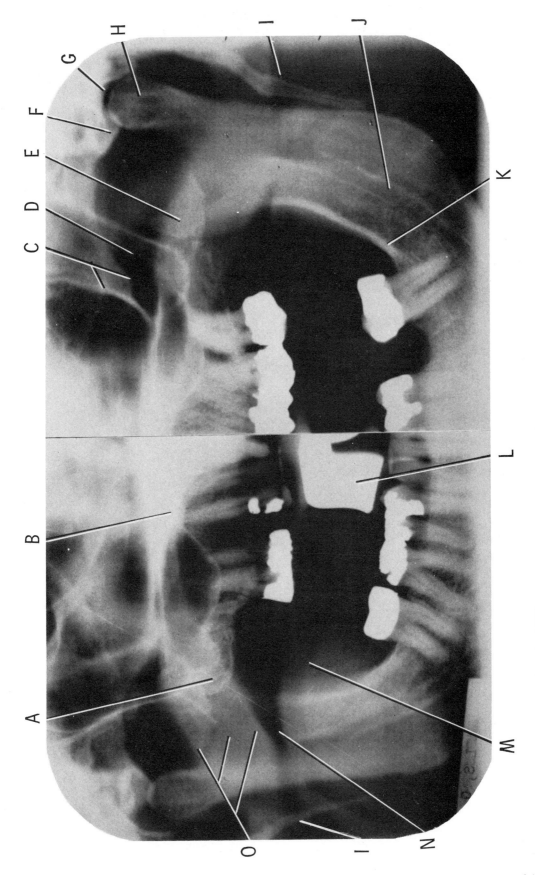

113

Plate 56     PANORAMIC VIEW (EDENTULOUS) _____

A. Coronoid process of mandible
B. Maxillary tuberosity
C. Nasal fossa
D. Nasal septum
E. Hard palate
F. Orbit
G. Maxillary sinus
H. Zygomatic arch
I. Articular eminence
J. Mandibular condyle
K. Cervical vertebrae
L. Facial artery notch
M. Mandibular canal
N. Plastic chin rest
O. Symphysis
P. Mental foramen
Q. Shadow of tongue
R. Angle of mandible
S. Pharynx
T. Mandibular foramen

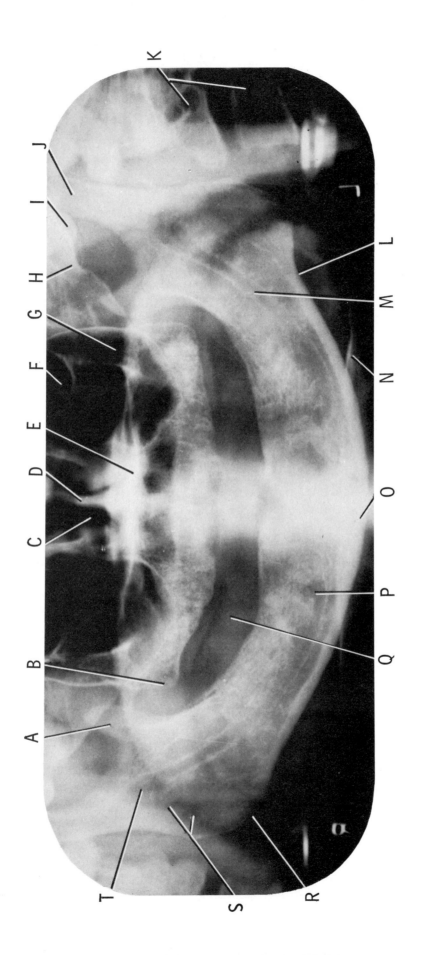

Plate 57     PANORAMIC VIEW  (CHERUBISM) _____

A.  Articular eminence
B.  Coronoid process of mandible
C.  Nasal concha
D.  Nasal septum
E.  Nasal fossa
F.  Maxillary sinus
G.  Symphysis
H.  Plastic chin rest
I.  Fibro-osseous lesion
J.  Angle of mandible
K.  Soft tissue of external ear (lobule)
L.  Cervical vertebra
M.  Mandibular condyle
N.  External auditory meatus
O.  Glenoid fossa

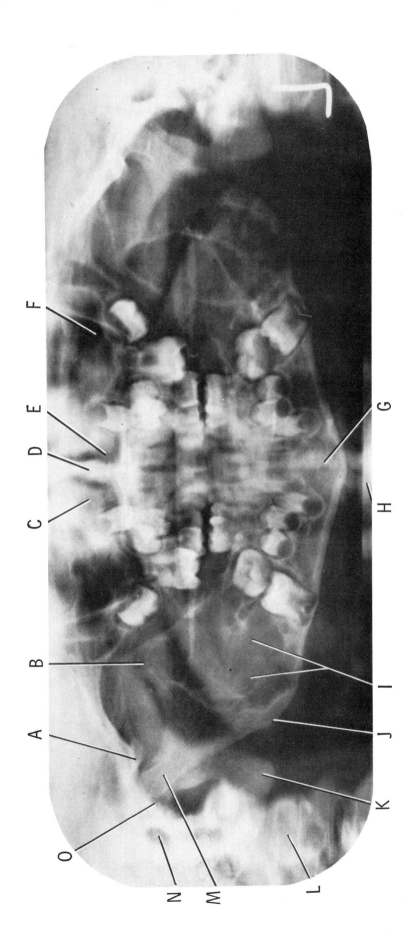

117

Plate 58    PANORAMIC VIEW _____

Film damaged by static electricity

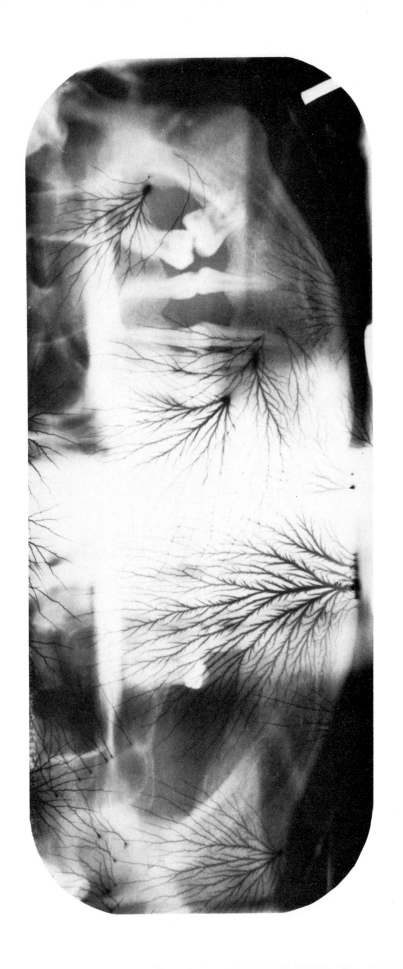

Plate 59    PANORAMIC VIEW _____

A.  Nasal fossa
B.  Nasal septum
C.  Hard palate
D.  Maxillary sinus
E.  Zygomatic arch
F.  Articular eminence
G.  Glenoid fossa
H.  Mandibular condyle
I.  Mental foramen
J.  Symphysis
K.  Mandibular canal
L.  Cervical vertebra
M.  Mandibular foramen
N.  Styloid process

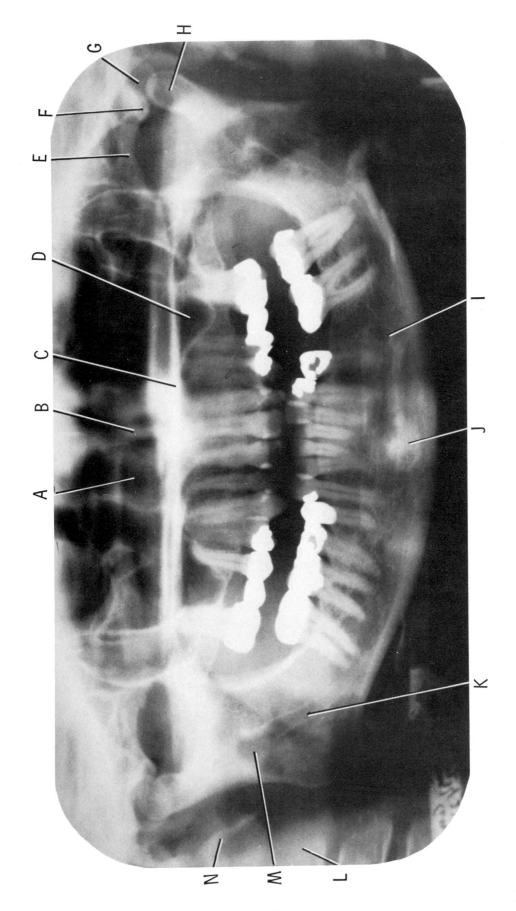

Plate 60    PANORAMIC VIEW _____

A.  Maxillary sinus
B.  Nasal fossa
C.  Hard palate
D.  Zygomatic arch
E.  Mandibular canal
F.  Oropharynx
G.  Symphysis
H.  External oblique ridge
I.  Soft palate

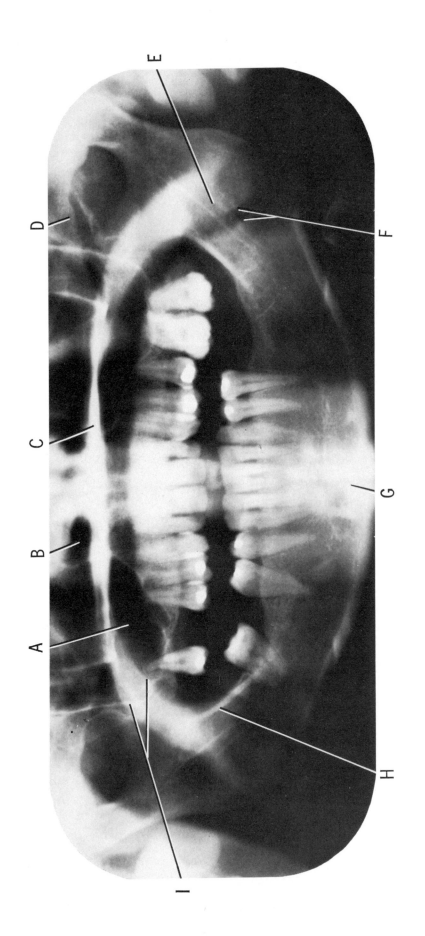

Plate 61      PANORAMIC VIEW (EDENTULOUS) _____

A. Mandibular notch
B. Nasal concha
C. Nasal septum
D. Nasal fossa
E. Hard palate
F. Articular eminence
G. Glenoid fossa
H. Mandibular condyle
I. External oblique ridge
J. Mental foramen
K. Shadow of ramus of opposite side

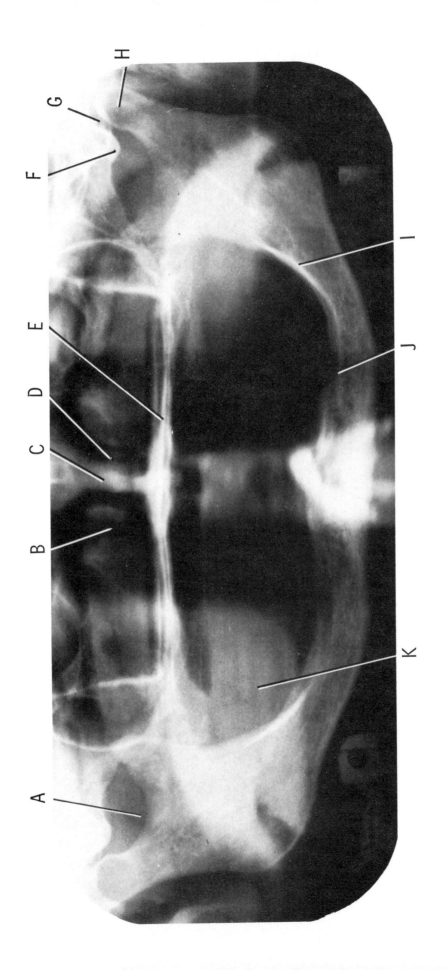

125

Plate 62   PANORAMIC VIEW

A. Maxillary sinus
B. Area of no radiation exposure
C. Nasal septum
D. Nasal fossa and concha
E. Hard palate
F. Plastic chin rest
G. Large carious lesion
H. Maxillary permanent lateral incisor
I. Maxillary permanent central incisor of opposite side
J. Carious lesion
K. Shadow of plastic chin rest of opposite side
L. Shadow of ramus of opposite side
M. Soft tissue of external ear (lobule)
N. External auditory meatus

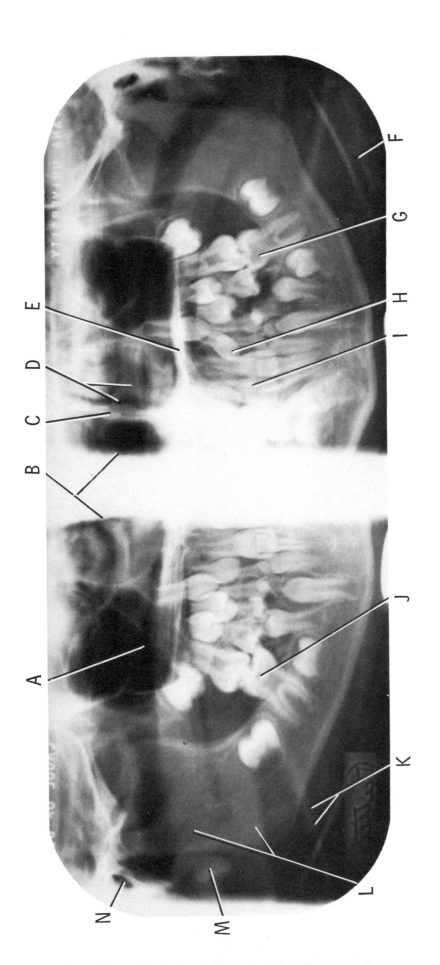

Plate 63    LATERAL HEADPLATE VIEW

A.    External cortical plate
B.    Internal cortical plate
C.    Coronal suture
D.    Artifact
E.    Anterior clinoid process
F.    Roof of orbit
G.    Nasal fossa
H.    Nasal bone
I.    Anterior nasal spine
J.    Developing mandibular permanent second molar in follicle
K.    Sphenoid sinus
L.    External auditory meatus
M.    Pituitary fossa in sella turcica
N.    Mastoid process
O.    Occipitomastoid suture
P.    Posterior clinoid process
Q.    Lambdoid suture
R.    Squamous suture

Plate 63    LATERAL  HEADPLATE  VIEW

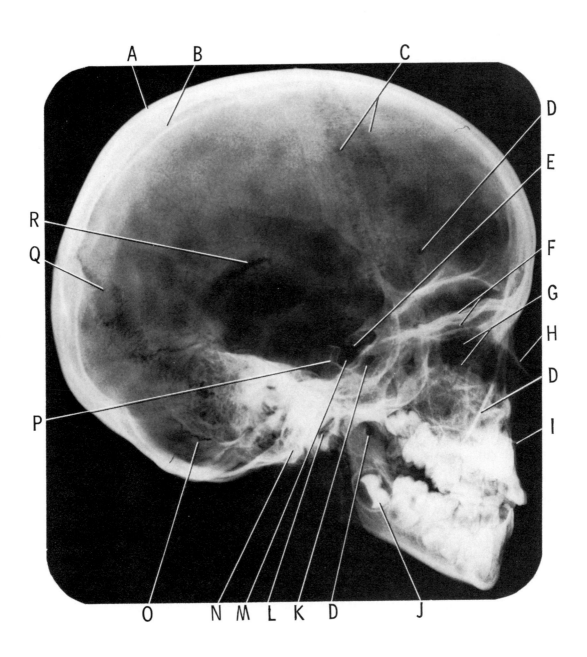

Plate 64    LATERAL HEADPLATE VIEW _____

| | |
|---|---|
| **A.** | Metal ear rod |
| **B.** | Pituitary fossa in sella turcica |
| **C.** | Roof of orbit |
| **D.** | Anterior clinoid process |
| **E.** | Frontal sinus |
| **F.** | Plastic orbital pointer |
| **G.** | Posterior clinoid process |
| **H.** | Sphenoid sinus |
| **I.** | Orbit |
| **J.** | Nasal fossa |
| **K.** | Anterior nasal spine |
| **L.** | Floor of nasal fossa |
| **M.** | Roof of maxillary sinus |
| **N.** | Maxillary sinus |

| | |
|---|---|
| **O.** | Posterior border of tongue |
| **P.** | Oropharynx |
| **Q.** | Hyoid bone |
| **R.** | Posterior pharyngeal wall |
| **S.** | Body of third cervical vertebra |
| **T.** | Body of fourth cervical vertebra |
| **U.** | Body of fifth cervical vertebra |
| **V.** | Body of axis |
| **W.** | Spinous processes of third, fourth and fifth cervical vertebrae |
| **X.** | Soft palate |
| **Y.** | Spinous process of axis |
| **Z.** | Spinous process of atlas |

| | |
|---|---|
| **a.** | Nasopharynx |
| **b.** | Odontoid process of axis |
| **c.** | Anterior tubercle of atlas |
| **d.** | Occipital eminence |

| | |
|---|---|
| **e.** | Occipital condyle |
| **f.** | Mastoid air cells |
| **g.** | Shadow of petrosal pyramid of temporal bone |

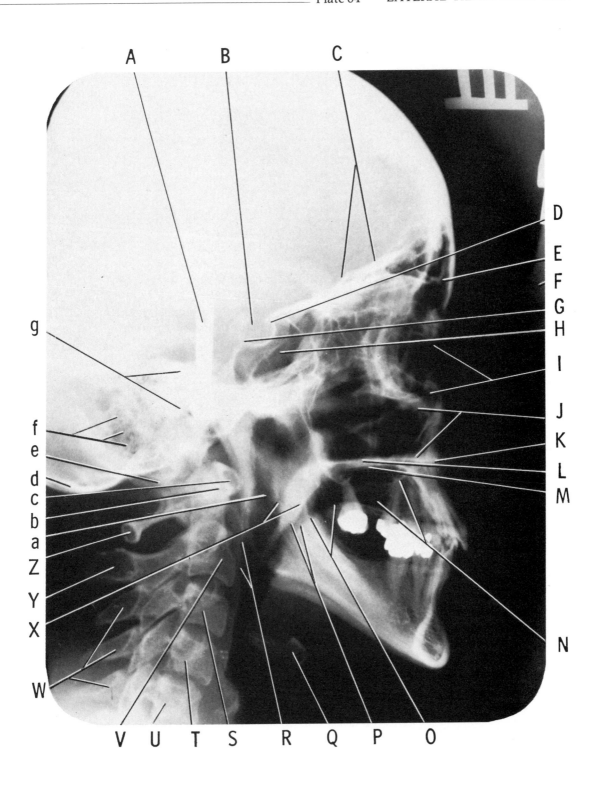

Plate 65    LATERAL HEADPLATE VIEW _____

A.  Coronal suture
B.  Inner cortical plate
C.  Outer cortical plate
D.  Roof of orbit
E.  Frontal sinus
F.  Orbit
G.  Sphenoid sinus
H.  Maxillary sinus superimposed over nasal fossa
I.  Radiopaque material painted on the dorsum of the tongue
J.  Lip of maxilla
K.  Lip of mandible
L.  Mandibular permanent first and second bicuspids
M.  Mandibular permanent first and second molars

N.  Unerupted mandibular permanent third molar
O.  Soft palate
P.  Hyoid bone
Q.  Oropharynx
R.  Nasopharynx
S.  Fourth cervical vertebra
T.  Third cervical vertebra
U.  Axis
V.  Atlas
W.  Pituitary fossa in sella turcica
X.  Mastoid air cells
Y.  Plastic ear rod and head holder
Z.  Posterior clinoid process

a.  Metal hairpins

Plate 65     LATERAL  HEADPLATE  VIEW

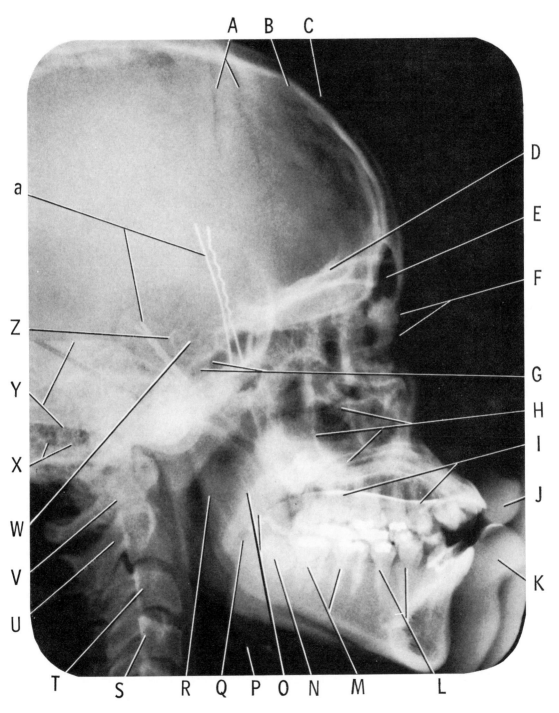

Plate 66    LATERAL HEADPLATE VIEW _____

| | | | |
|---|---|---|---|
| A. | Patient identification plate | N. | Maxillary permanent first bicuspid |
| B. | Inner cortical plate | O. | Maxillary permanent second bicuspid |
| C. | Outer cortical plate | P. | Maxillary permanent first molar |
| D. | Posterior clinoid process | Q. | Maxillary primary molars |
| E. | Pituitary fossa in sella turcica | R. | Mandibular permanent first bicuspid |
| F. | Roof of orbit | S. | Mandibular primary second molar |
| G. | Anterior clinoid process | T. | Mandibular permanent second bicuspid |
| H. | Frontal sinus | | |
| I. | Sphenoid sinus | U. | Mandibular permanent first molar |
| J. | Orbit | V. | Maxillary permanent second molar |
| K. | Maxillary sinus superimposed over nasal fossa | W. | Mandibular permanent second molar |
| | | X. | Hyoid bone |
| L. | Hard palate | Y. | Oropharynx |
| M. | Unerupted maxillary permanent cuspid | Z. | Soft palate |

_____

| | | | |
|---|---|---|---|
| a. | Nasopharynx | g. | Odontoid process of axis |
| b. | Pharyngeal wall | h. | Mastoid air cells |
| c. | Fourth cervical vertebra | i. | Outer cortical plate of occipital bone |
| d. | Third cervical vertebra | j. | Inner cortical plate of occipital bone |
| e. | Axis | k. | Plastic ear rod and head holder |
| f. | Atlas | l. | Lambdoid suture |

Plate 66    LATERAL  HEADPLATE  VIEW

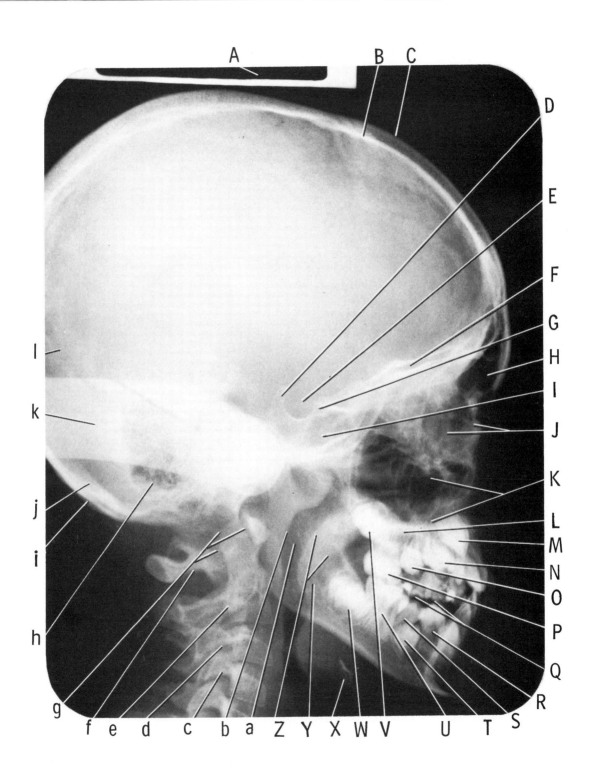

Plate 67     POSTEROANTERIOR HEADPLATE VIEW _____

A.  Sagittal suture
B.  Coronal suture
C.  Greater wing of sphenoid
D.  Superior border of orbit
E.  Nasal septum
F.  Nasal concha
G.  Primary central incisor of maxilla
H.  Unerupted permanent first molar of mandible
I.  Angle of mandible
J.  Inferior border of mandible
K.  Shadow of cervical vertebrae
L.  Primary cuspid of mandible
M.  Unerupted mandibular permanent central incisor
N.  Unerupted mandibular permanent lateral incisor
O.  Unerupted mandibular permanent cuspid
P.  Mandibular primary left central incisor
Q.  Mandibular primary right central incisor
R.  Unerupted maxillary permanent central incisor
S.  Unerupted maxillary permanent first molar
T.  Maxillary sinus
U.  Foramen rotundum
V.  Crista galli

Plate 67    POSTEROANTERIOR  HEADPLATE  VIEW

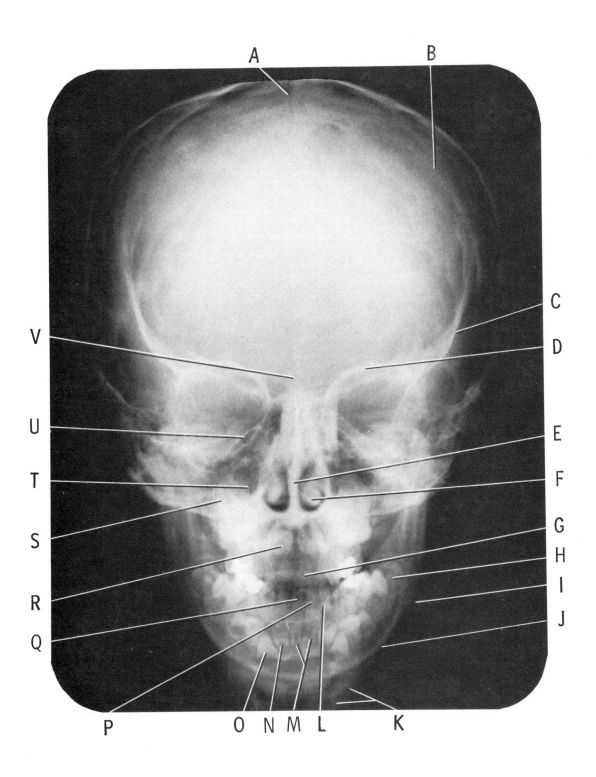

Plate 68     POSTEROANTERIOR  HEADPLATE  VIEW  _____

A.     Midsagittal suture
B.     Frontal sinus
C.     Plastic head positioner
D.     Mastoid air cells
E.     Nasal septum
F.     Nasal concha
G.     Anterior nasal spine
H.     Unerupted maxillary permanent second molar
I.     Unerupted mandibular permanent second molar
J.     Maxillary permanent central incisors
K.     Mandibular permanent central incisors
L.     Mandibular permanent lateral incisor
M.     Unerupted mandibular permanent cuspid
N.     Mandibular permanent first bicuspid
O.     Angle of mandible
P.     Neck of ramus of mandible
Q.     Maxillary sinus
R.     Petrous portion of temporal bone
S.     Orbit

Plate 68    POSTEROANTERIOR  HEADPLATE  VIEW

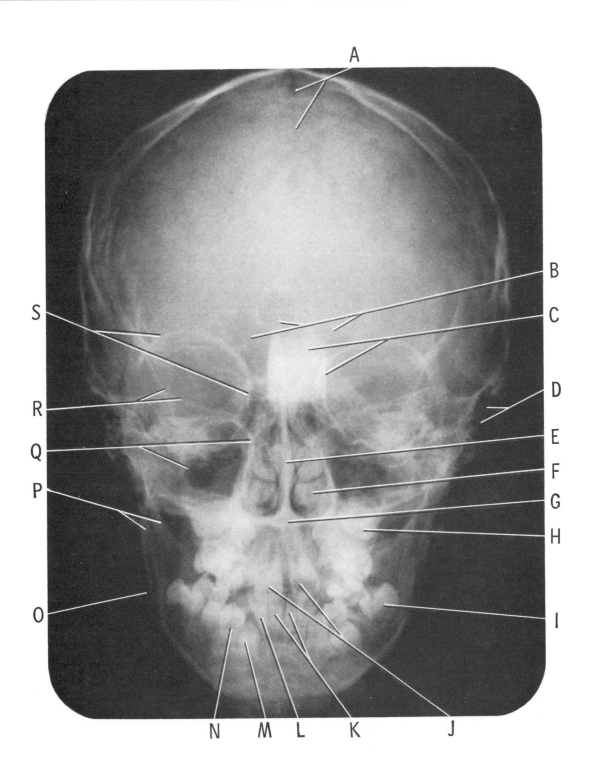

Plate 69     WATERS' SINUS HEADPLATE VIEW _____

A.     Frontal sinus
B.     Orbit
C.     Nasal septum
D.     Nasal conchae
E.     Maxillary sinus
F.     Zygomatic arch
G.     Anterior teeth of mandible
H.     Odontoid process of axis
I.     Foramen magnum
J.     Inferior border of mandible
K.     Posterior border of ramus of mandible
L.     Foramen rotundum

Plate 69    WATERS' SINUS HEADPLATE VIEW

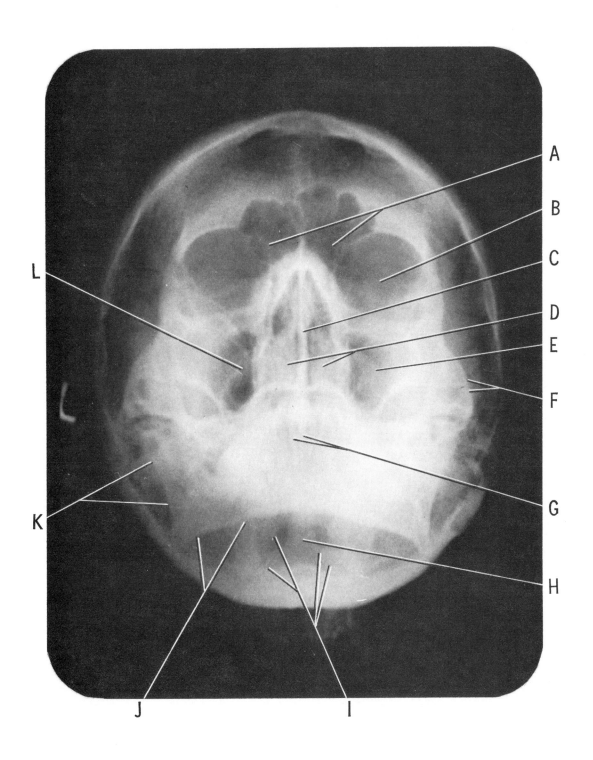

Plate 70      TEMPOROMANDIBULAR  JOINT  VIEW  (UPDEGRAVE) _____

A.  Open position
B.  Rest position
C.  Closed position
D.  Glenoid fossa
E.  Cranium interior
F.  Head of mandibular condyle
G.  Articular eminence
H.  External auditory meatus

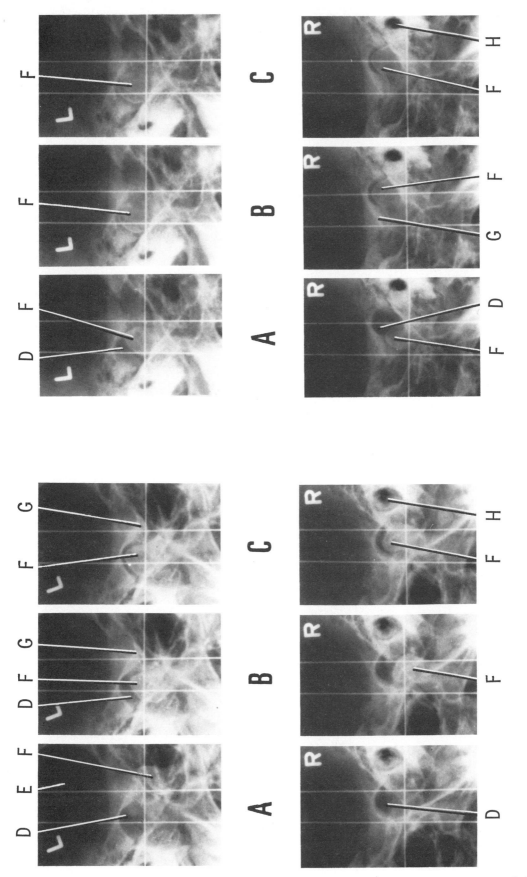

Plate 71    TEMPOROMANDIBULAR JOINT VIEW (TRANSORBITAL) _____

A.    Zygomatic arch
B.    Medial third of head of condyle
C.    Lateral third of head of condyle
D.    Neck of condyle
E.    Styloid process
F.    Mastoid process

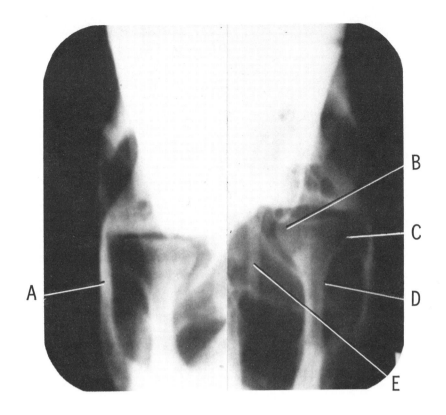

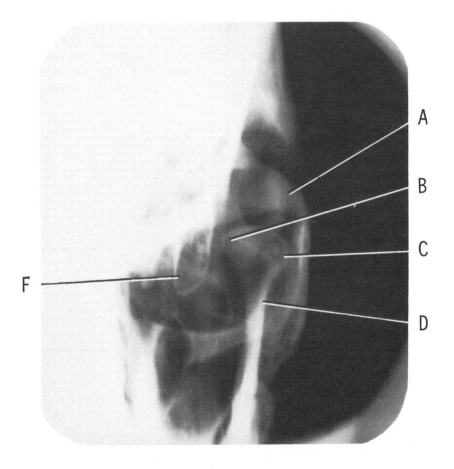

Plate 72     TEMPOROMANDIBULAR JOINT VIEW _____

**A.**     The single arrowhead indicates an area of agenesis of the mandibular condyle. The double arrows indicate a normal mandibular condyle on the opposite side.

**B.**     This is a transpharyngeal view of the mandibular condyle. The single arrow indicates the location of the condyle; the arrowhead points to the sella turcica. The radiolucency inferior and anterior to the sella is the sphenoid sinus.

Plate 72    TEMPOROMANDIBULAR JOINT VIEW

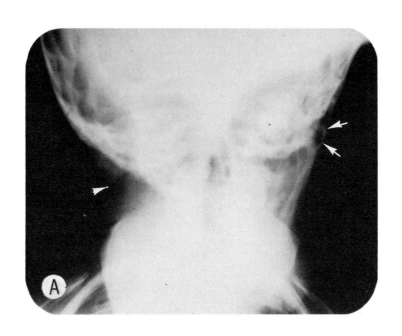

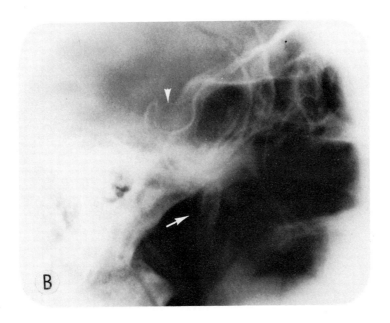

Plate 73    TEMPOROMANDIBULAR JOINT VIEW _____

**A.**    This is a straight lateral tomogram of the right condyle of a 26-year-old patient.

**B.**    This is a corrected axis tomogram of the same condyle. It displays a more accurate radiographic view of this condyle.

(Tomograms courtesy of Dr. A. Sondhi.)

Plate 73    TEMPOROMANDIBULAR JOINT VIEW

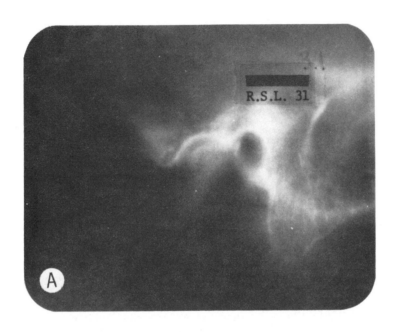

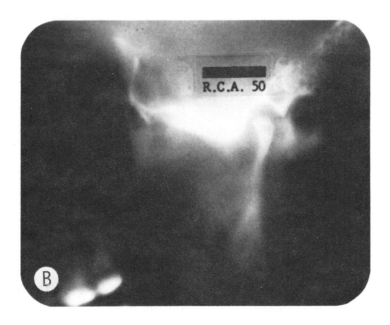

Plate 74     TEMPOROMANDIBULAR JOINT VIEW _____

**A.**    This right corrected axis tomogram reveals a flat condyle (arrowheads). There was pain in the temporomandibular joint.

**B.**    This is a right corrected axis tomogram showing a cystic erosive change (arrow) in the condyle. The patient was a 50-year-old woman with a history of dull pain in the temporomandibular joint.

(Tomograms courtesy of Dr. A. Sondhi.)

Plate 74    TEMPOROMANDIBULAR JOINT VIEW

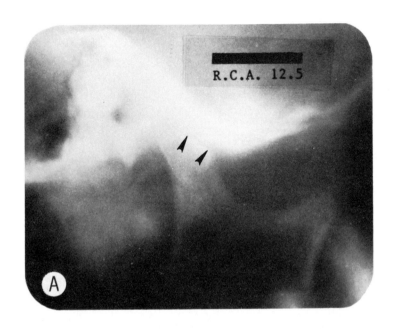

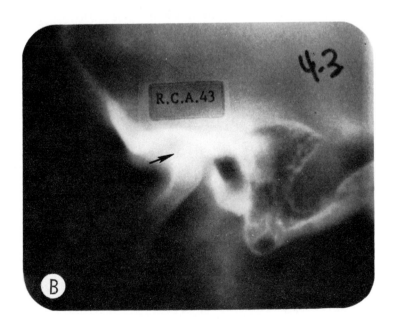

Plate 75     TEMPOROMANDIBULAR JOINT VIEW _____

**A.** The condyle shown here was fixed in a dislocated position (not in the glenoid fossa) following a subcondylar osteotomy. The fossa had calcified during the ensuing years (arrowheads), with some accommodation to this condition by the patient but with persistent temporomandibular joint pain as well.

**B.** In this case, diagnosed as degenerative osteoarthritic change and loss of joint space (in a 49-year-old woman who experienced pain in the temporomandibular joint), there is a bone spur on the condyle (arrow). The external auditory meatus (1) and the mastoid air cells (2) are identified.

(Tomograms courtesy of Dr. A. Sondhi.)

Plate 75    TEMPOROMANDIBULAR JOINT VIEW

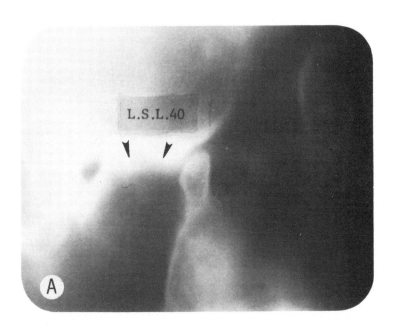

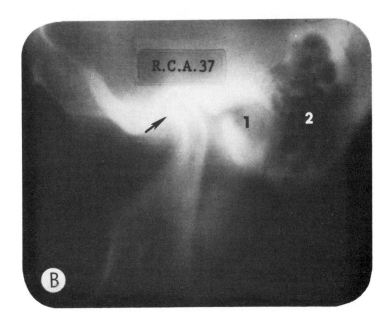

Plate 76    TEMPOROMANDIBULAR JOINT VIEW _____

**A.**    Corrected axis radiograph showing left condyle position (arrowhead) at physiologic rest.

**B.**    Corrected axis radiograph showing left condyle position (arrowhead) with maximum intercuspation.

**C.**    Corrected axis radiograph showing limited translation of left condyle (arrowhead) with maximum opening.

(Radiographs courtesy of Dr. J. Green.)

Plate 76    TEMPOROMANDIBULAR JOINT VIEW

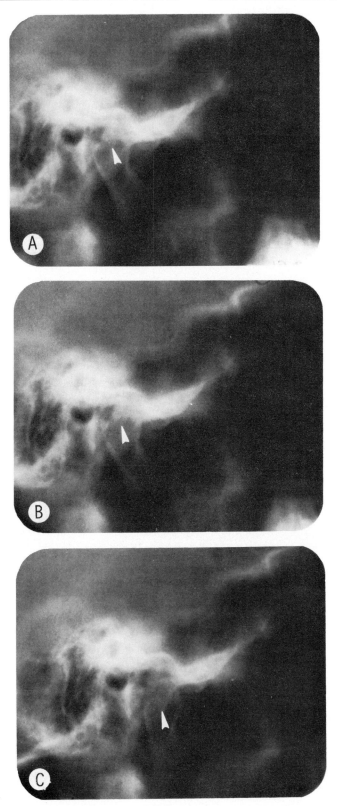

Plate 77     TEMPOROMANDIBULAR JOINT VIEW _____

**A, B, C.**     Corrected axis tomograms showing decreased joint space and posterior positioning of left condyle (arrowheads) due to anteriorly displaced meniscus.

(Tomograms courtesy of Dr. J. Green.)

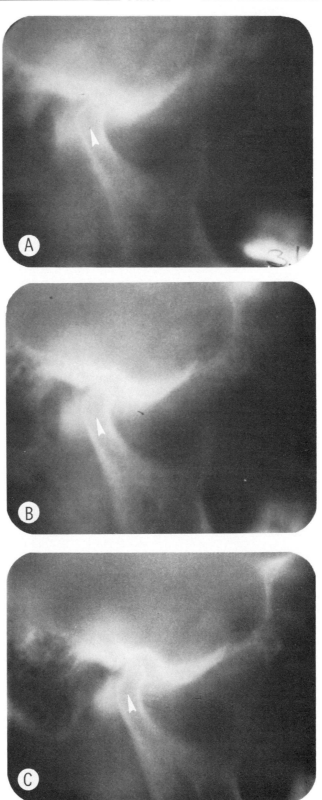

Plate 78     TEMPOROMANDIBULAR JOINT VIEW _____

 

A.   Corrected axis radiograph showing right condyle position at physiologic rest (osteophytic spur [arrowhead] visible on anterior surface of condyle).

B.   Corrected axis radiograph showing right condyle position at maximum intercuspation (osteophytic spur [arrowhead] visible on anterior surface of condyle).

C.   Corrected axis radiograph showing limited translation of right condyle with maximum opening (osteophytic spur [arrowhead] visible on anterior surface of condyle).

(Radiographs courtesy of Dr. J. Green.)

Plate 78    TEMPOROMANDIBULAR JOINT VIEW

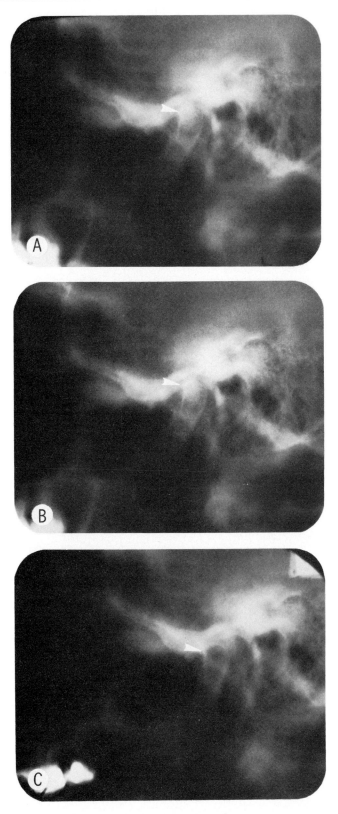

Plate 79    TEMPOROMANDIBULAR JOINT VIEW _____

**A, B.**    Corrected axis tomograms showing osteophytic spur (arrowheads) on right condyle, indicating degenerative joint disease (osteoarthritis).

(Tomograms courtesy of Dr. J. Green.)

Plate 79    TEMPOROMANDIBULAR JOINT VIEW

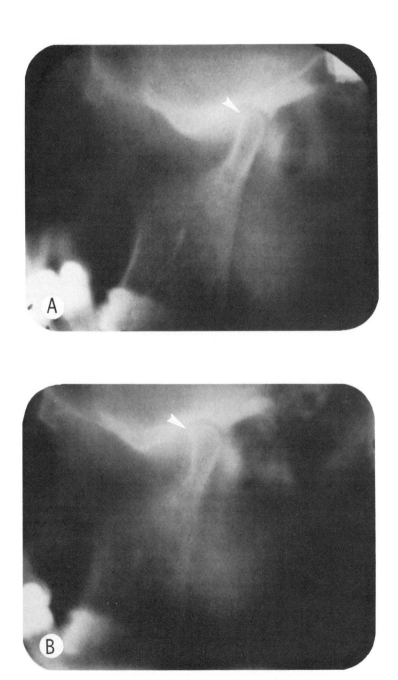

# section three

## FILM ARTIFACTS AND TECHNICAL ERRORS

Plate 80    ELONGATED IMAGE; RADIOPAQUE IMAGE; FILM PLACEMENT _____

A.    Due to a reduced positive vertical angulation, these teeth appear elongated. This effect is the opposite of foreshortening.

B.    The operator forgot to remove the patient's maxillary gold partial denture. The large radiopaque area represents the image of the denture.

C.    When the film was placed in the mouth, it was not positioned far down enough to include the roots of the teeth. If a film holder is used, it is likely that this will not occur.

D.    This film was curved when the patient closed down on the film holder. The radiopaque image at the top of this film is that of the metal film holder.

Plate 80     ELONGATED IMAGE; RADIOPAQUE IMAGE; FILM PLACEMENT

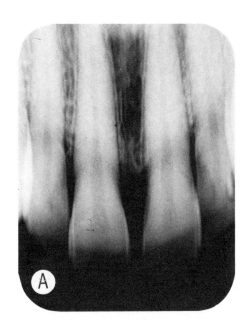

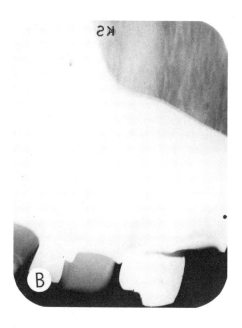

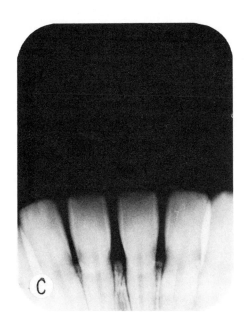

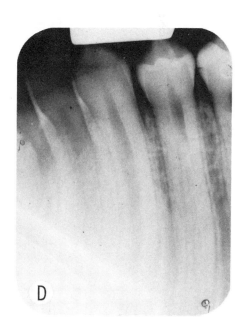

Plate 81     REVERSED FILM; CONE CUT; EYEGLASS ARTIFACT _____

A.     When placed in the patient's mouth, this film was reversed. The film's tab was facing the lingual aspect of the teeth. The "tire track" design on the film is actually the image of the lead foil that is in the film packet. Radiation has passed through the lead foil, not only leaving its impression on the film but also causing the radiograph to appear too light.

B.     The same thing has happened to this radiograph. The lead foil design looks a little different but it is still due to the film's being placed backwards in the patient's mouth.

C.     The crowns have been obliterated by a cone cut.

D.     The operator failed to remove the patient's eyeglasses, accounting for the large radiopaque area over the apices of the premolars.

Plate 81     REVERSED FILM; CONE CUT; EYEGLASS  ARTIFACT

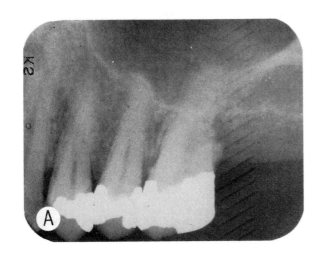

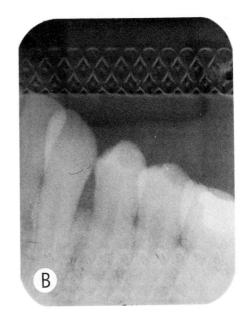

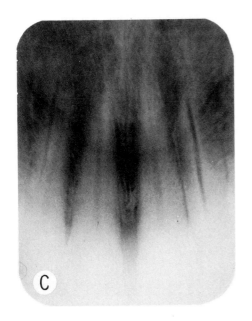

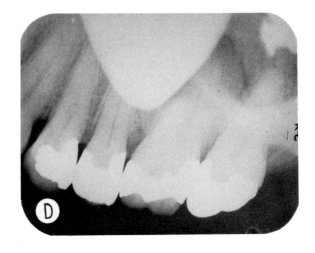

Plate 82     EXPOSURE PROBLEMS; MOTION;————————————————————
                 DOUBLE IMAGE;
                 FORESHORTENED IMAGES

A.     Exposing a radiograph to more radiation than is needed (overexposure) will cause the film to appear too dark after development. That is probably the problem with this radiograph. This could also happen if the film is developed too long or if too high a kilovoltage is used.

B.     The appearance of motion in this radiograph might be due to film motion, patient motion, or excessive x-ray cone motion during the time the film was exposed to radiation.

C.     You are seeing double in this radiograph. The operator accidentally exposed this radiograph twice, thus producing two sets of dental images.

D.     These images are foreshortened. Excessive positive vertical angulation of the x-ray cone produces this effect; insufficient positive vertical angulation causes elongation.

Plate 82    EXPOSURE PROBLEMS; MOTION;
DOUBLE IMAGE;
FORESHORTENED IMAGES

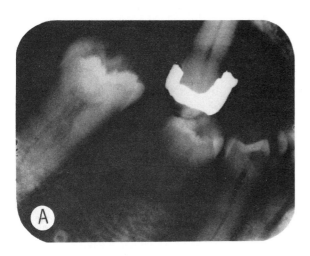

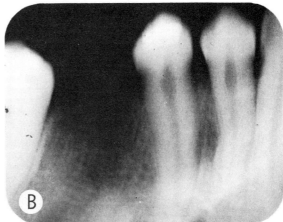

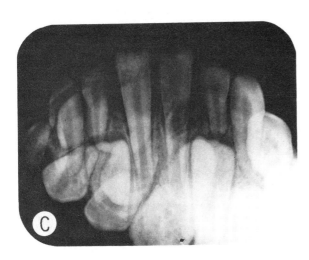

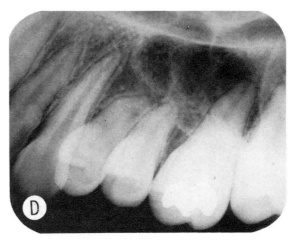

Plate 83     PROCESSING AND POSITIONING
ERRORS; CONE CUT;
OVERLAPPING

A.     Superimposed over the mesial root of the first molar is a chemical artifact, not a dental lesion. This is due to dried fixer that had remained on the film hanger clip and contaminated the film during development. Film hangers should be thoroughly washed in water before they are used.

B.     When film is improperly positioned in the patient's mouth, a poor radiograph results. The film should have been placed posteriorly enough for the third molar to be entirely visible.

C.     This is classified as a posterior cone cut because the cone cut is posterior to the most distal molar.

D.     If horizontal angulation of the x-ray cone had been properly set, overlapping of these interproximals would likely not have occurred.

Plate 83     PROCESSING  AND  POSITIONING
ERRORS;  CONE  CUT;
OVERLAPPING

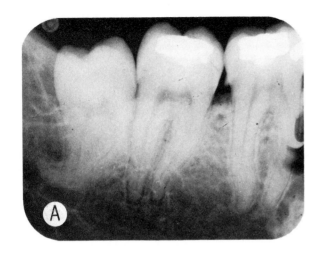

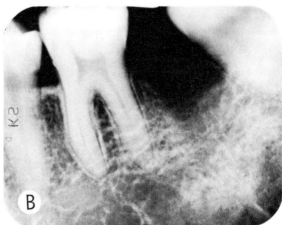

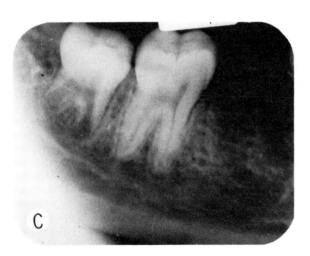

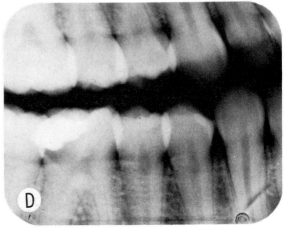

Plate 84     PROCESSING ERRORS; UNAVOIDABLE FILM ARTIFACTS  _____

**A.**   This film was placed in developer at an elevated temperature. When removed from the developer the film was allowed to dry before placement in rinse water. Dried developer spots now mottle the film.

**B.**   The white streaks on this film are due to fixer solution contamination.

**C.**   The white vertical lines seen along the edges of this film are due to folding of the film packet. Folding is sometimes necessary if the film is too large for the patient's mouth.

**D.**   The film emulsion has been scratched. When the film is processed in the manual processor, the soft emulsion is easily scratched in the processing tanks.

Plate 84    PROCESSING ERRORS; UNAVOIDABLE FILM ARTIFACTS

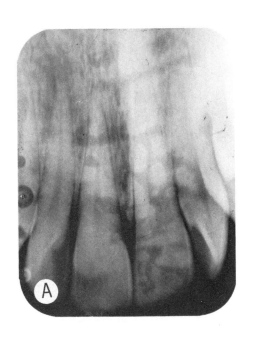

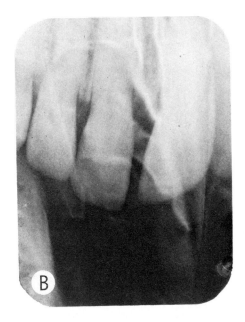

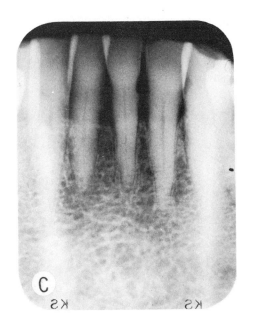

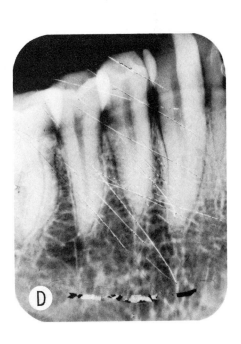

Plate 85     OVERLAPPING; CONE CUTS _____

A.     Overlapping of tooth contacts interferes with proper interpretation of interproximal details.
B.     An anterior film cone cut is a technical error.
C.     Improper horizontal angulation of the x-ray equipment cone can cause image overlapping like that seen in this film.
D.     This is commonly called a superior film cone cut.

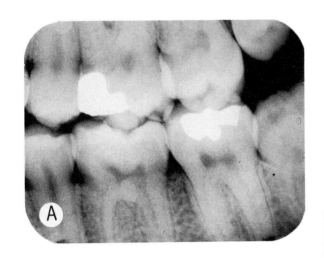

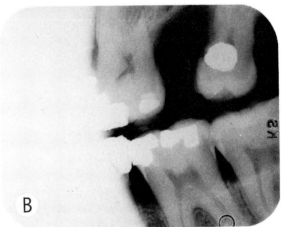

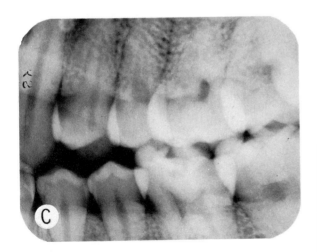

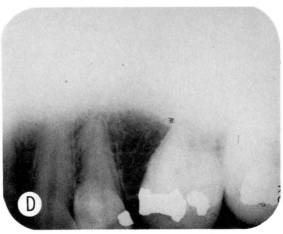

Plate 86     DOUBLE AND REVERSED IMAGE; DEVELOPER ARTIFACT _____

**A.**     Occlusal films are sometimes double-exposed. The film packet was also placed backwards in the patient's mouth. Notice the "tire tracks" from the lead foil backing in the film packet.

**B.**     The black spots on the film are developer solution stains. There also appear to be two supernumerary teeth developing in the palate.

Plate 86    DOUBLE AND REVERSED IMAGE; DEVELOPER ARTIFACT

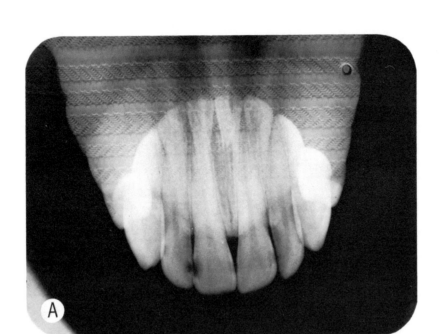

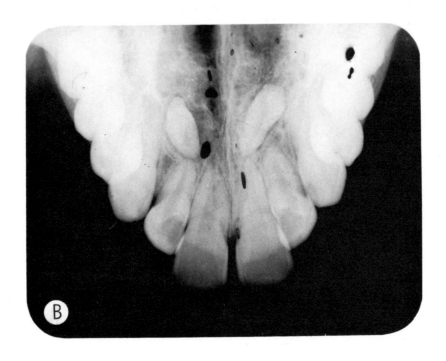

Plate 87    OPAQUE ARTIFACTS (PROCESSING ERROR) _____

The operator did not remove the inner paper wrapping surrounding the film. When the film was processed, air was trapped between the film and paper surfaces. Those areas that were not properly developed appear as opaque artifacts.

Plate 87     OPAQUE ARTIFACTS (PROCESSING ERROR)

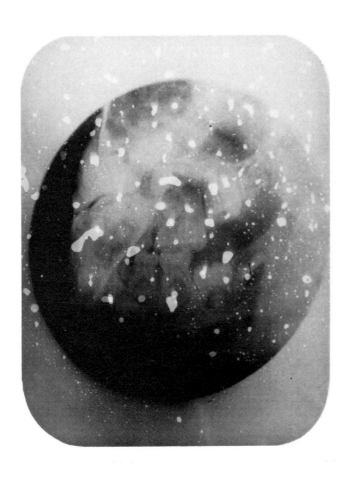

Plate 88     PROCESSING ERRORS _____

**A.**     A fingerprint can be seen over the roots of the premolars. The operator's hands had been exposed to fluoride solution and were not washed before developing this film. Developer solution could cause this same artifact.

**B.**     This is one of two films that adhered to each other during the developing and fixing process. The film cannot be improved, as the emulsion has been damaged.

**C.**     During processing of this film, another film overlapped it. This is the reason you see a line through the molars. Fixer was accidentally spilled on this film before developing. This is evidenced by the opaque spots on the mesial root apices of the first and second molars.

**D.**     When developer solution is smeared on a film prior to development, this is the usual result.

Plate 88    PROCESSING ERRORS

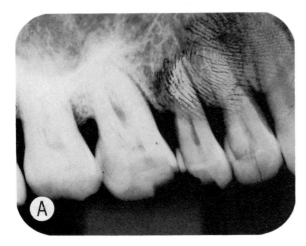

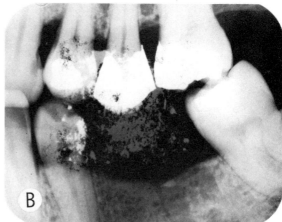

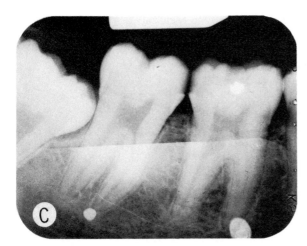

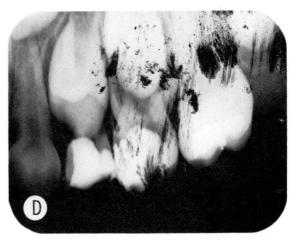

Plate 89    CHEMICAL SPILLS; PACKAGING ARTIFACT _____

A.    There are black dots on this film. They were caused by developer solution accidentally spilled on the film before developing.

B.    The white images that appear on the roots of these teeth are drops of fixer solution, which was accidentally spilled on the film before developing.

C.    The large black area on this film was caused by developer solution splashed on the film before developing.

D.    This is an unusual packaging artifact that is very likely caused by the inner black paper covering the film.

Plate 89    CHEMICAL SPILLS; PACKAGING ARTIFACT

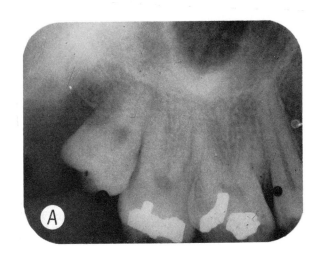

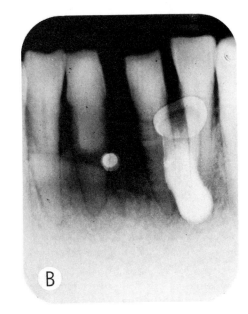

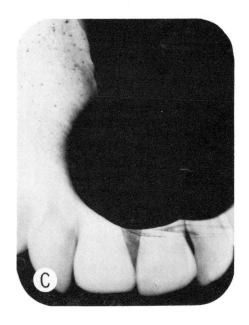

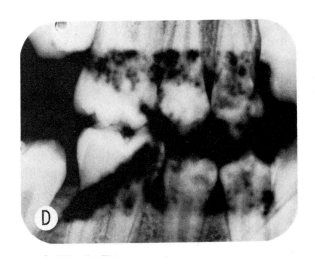

# section four

## ITEMS COMMONLY SEEN IN DENTAL RADIOGRAPHS

Plate 90     PORCELAIN; METAL ARTIFACTS ⎯⎯⎯⎯⎯⎯⎯⎯⎯⎯⎯⎯⎯⎯

**A.**     The porcelain sanitary pontic shows up well on this radiograph. The radiopaque spot under the pontic is most likely silver alloy.

**B.**     If you look closely at the radiopaque object you can recognize the tip of a dental bur.

**C.**     All of the radiopaque spots represent metal fragments from a shotgun injury. The fragments are in the patient's cheek.

**D.**     The radiopaque object superimposed over the second molar is a metal clasp that is attached to an acrylic partial denture (the acrylic partial denture does not show radiographically).

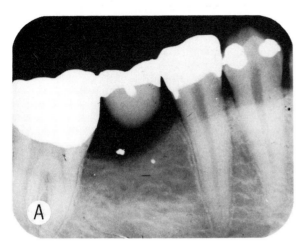

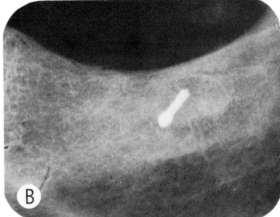

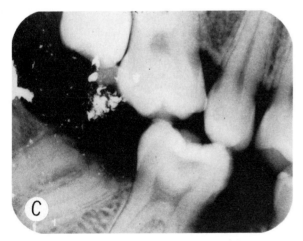

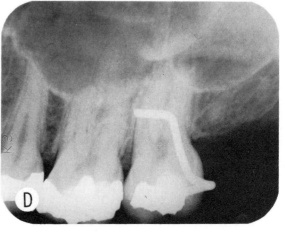

Plate 91     IMPLANT; CANTILEVERED BRIDGE; _____
             DILACERATED ROOTS;
             RESORBED ROOTS

 

**A.**     This is a blade implant used as an abutment for a bridge.
**B.**     This four-unit bridge has a distal cantilevered unit.
**C.**     The second and third molars have roots that have undergone severe dilaceration.
**D.**     The distal root of the first molar has resorbed, and it appears that the pulp chamber and canals have calcified.

Plate 91    IMPLANT; CANTILEVERED BRIDGE;
DILACERATED ROOTS;
RESORBED ROOTS

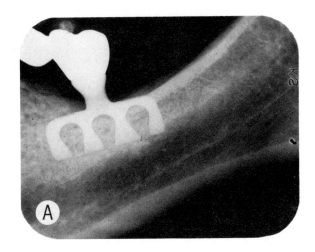

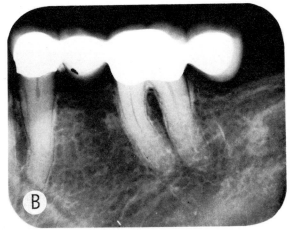

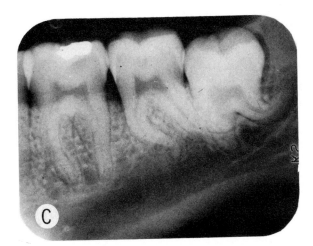

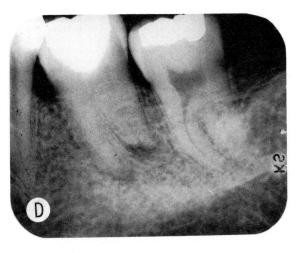

Plate 92    PINS; POST AND CORE; RETROGRADE ALLOYS _____

A.    A stainless steel pin was placed in the second molar. It is a mystery why the pin was placed.

B.    The gold post and core restoration was too broad. It also does not follow the canal, which was endodontically treated. Oxyphosphate cement used to fix the post and core restoration is seen leaking laterally through the fractured portion of the tooth.

C.    The retrograde silver alloy missed its mark at the apex of the right central incisor.

D.    The endodontic treatment in the first premolar looks good but something went wrong with the attempted retrograde silver alloy restoration.

Plate 92    PINS; POST AND CORE; RETROGRADE ALLOYS

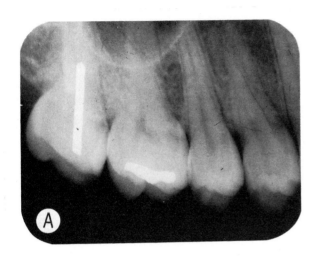

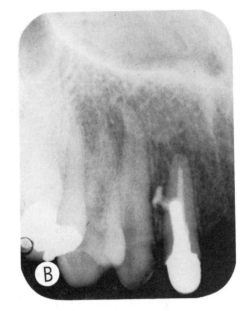

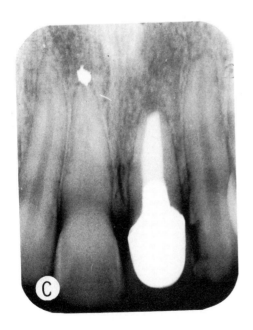

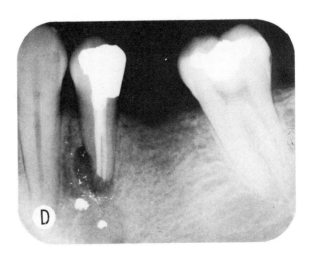

Plate 93    UNUSUAL FINDINGS; CALCIFIED PULP_____
            CHAMBER; RADIOLUCENCIES;
            STABILIZER PIN

A.    The facial and lingual surfaces of the appliance cemented in the root canals of these teeth were covered with a resin material. The dark radiolucent areas surrounding the apices of the teeth indicate loss of bone, a pathological development resulting from infection of the teeth.

B.    The cuspid demonstrates no pulp chamber. Diffuse calcification is a good description of this condition.

C.    The lingual access opening into the pulp chamber of the left central incisor is particularly evident from the large radiolucency in the crown.

D.    An endodontic stabilizer pin was used to anchor this tooth root in the bone.

Plate 93    UNUSUAL FINDINGS; CALCIFIED PULP
CHAMBER; RADIOLUCENCIES;
STABILIZER PIN

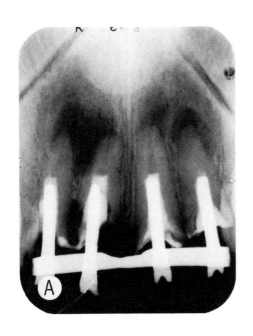

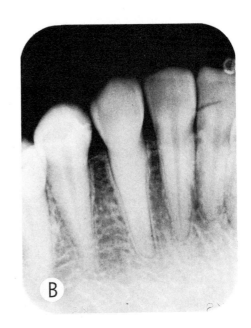

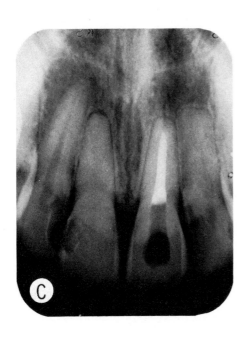

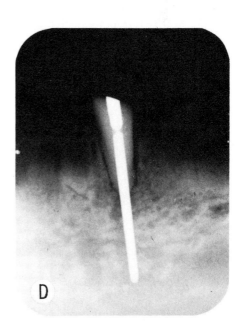

Plate 94    RESTORATIONS; RECURRENT CARIES; IMPEDED PREMOLAR ERUPTION _____

**A.**    A silver alloy restoration was placed in the first molar. Recurrent caries is evident. The radiopaque line just superior to the pulp chamber is secondary dentin.

**B.**    Reinforcing pins were placed in the right lateral incisor and both central incisors. They were used to reinforce their respective resin restorations. There is a large pathosis apical to the left lateral incisor, which has been endodontically treated and then fitted with a gold post and core.

**C.**    The lateral incisor has a poorly crafted retrograde silver alloy restoration.

**D.**    The second premolar is not likely to erupt normally. There is a copper band located just occlusal to the second premolar. You can barely see the remnants of the second primary molar inside the copper band.

Plate 94    RESTORATIONS; RECURRENT CARIES; IMPEDED PREMOLAR ERUPTION

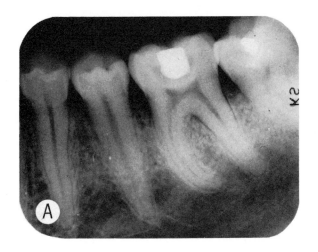

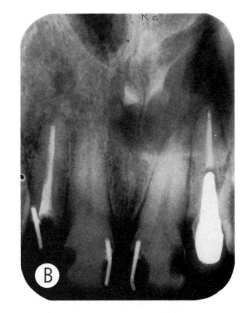

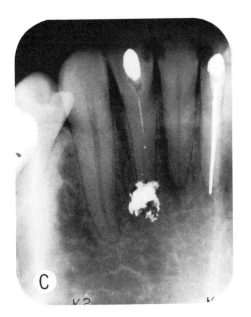

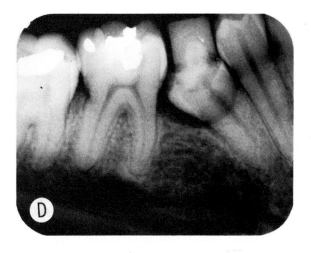

Plate 95     MUCOCELE; SUPERNUMERARY _____
TOOTH; MICRODONT;
EXTRUDED TEETH

**A.**     The semicircular gray area in the maxillary sinus is a mucocele. The
more radiopaque object at the top of the film is the zygomatic process.

**B.**     Between the roots of the maxillary second premolar and molar is a
developing supernumerary tooth.

**C.**     Just distal to the molar is a microdont.

**D.**     These teeth are extruded (over-erupted). They have no opposing teeth
in the mandible. Note the calculus between the molars.

Plate 95     MUCOCELE; SUPERNUMERARY
TOOTH; MICRODONT;
EXTRUDED TEETH

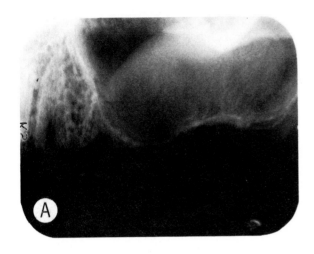

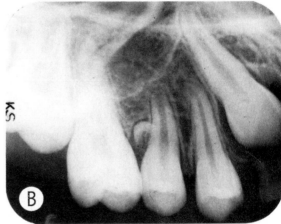

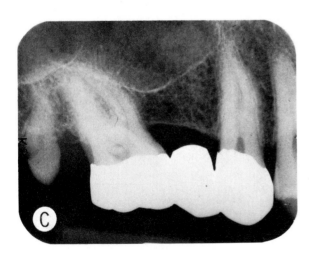

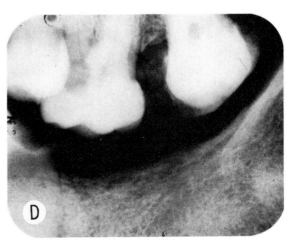

Plate 96      METALLIC ARTIFACTS _____

 

**A.**   It appears that some silver alloy has become wedged between the crown of the horizontal molar and the distal root of the erect molar.

**B.**   A reinforcing pin has accidentally penetrated through the mesial-cervical aspect of the maxillary second premolar.

**C.**   The radiopaque material just distal to the distal root of the second molar is a wire used to reduce a bone fracture.

**D.**   That radiopaque object in the bone is a piece of metal. No one seems to know how it got there.

Plate 96     METALLIC ARTIFACTS

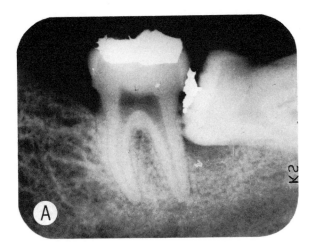

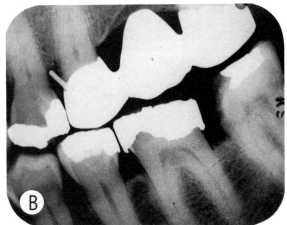

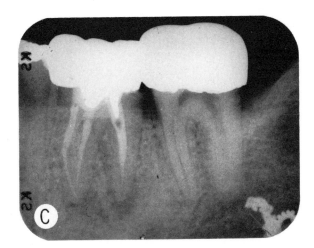

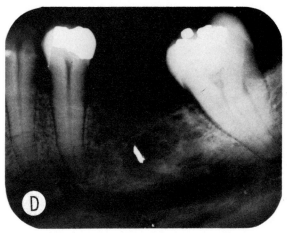

Plate 97       DENS IN DENTE; CALCIFIED PULP CHAMBER_____
AND CANAL; LINGUAL FORAMEN AND
CANAL; CEMENTOMA

 **A.** The lateral incisor has a developmental defect called dens invaginatus (dens in dente).

 **B.** Radiographically neither the pulp chamber nor the canal is revealed in the cuspid. Calcific metamorphosis has closed the pulp chamber and canal.

 **C.** There are no permanent lateral incisors. Note the lingual foramen and the lingual canal.

 **D.** These teeth were vital. The apical radiolucency with a calcified area in the center is periapical cemental dysplasia (cementoma).

Plate 97     DENS IN DENTE; CALCIFIED PULP CHAMBER
AND CANAL; LINGUAL FORAMEN AND
CANAL; CEMENTOMA

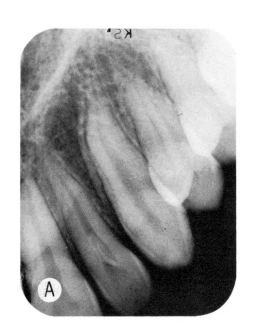

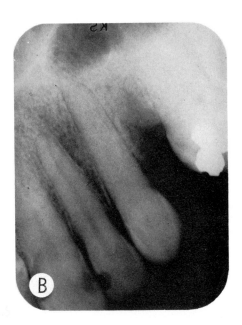

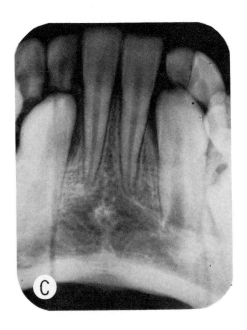

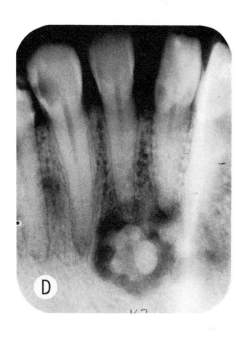

Plate 98     EXTRACTION SITE; CHANGES IN _____
LAMINA DURA; RUBBER-BASE
MATERIAL

A.     The extraction site of the second premolar is evident. The radiopaque lamina dura is distinct.

B.     The same extraction site has almost completely calcified several months later. The lamina dura is no longer distinct.

C.     The second premolar has been prepared for a full-crown restoration. A rubber-base elastic material was used to make an impression of the tooth preparation.

D.     Just distal to the prepared tooth is a radiopaque object that actually was a piece of the rubber-base material used to make an impression of the tooth preparation. The material appeared to leak into the gingival sulcus. It was removed without any postoperative problem.

Plate 98    EXTRACTION SITE; CHANGES IN
LAMINA DURA; RUBBER-BASE
MATERIAL

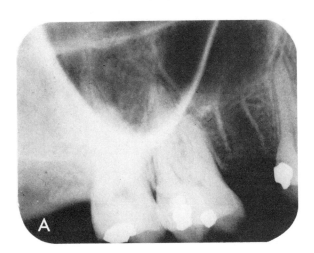

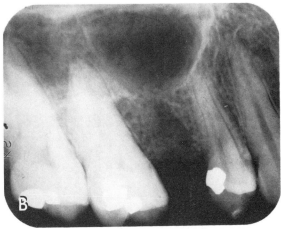

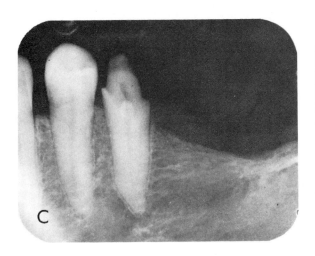

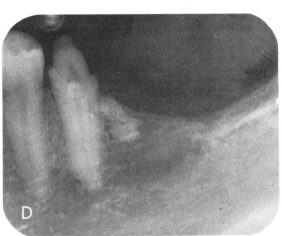

Plate 99       TAURODONT; CHRONIC DIFFUSE SCLEROSING OSTEOMYELITIS _____

 

**A.**       Both of these radiographs are from the same patient. The teeth demonstrate the typical form of taurodonts (or taurodontism).

**B.**       Both radiographs are from the same patient and demonstrate chronic diffuse sclerosing osteomyelitis.

Plate 99     TAURODONT; CHRONIC DIFFUSE SCLEROSING OSTEOMYELITIS

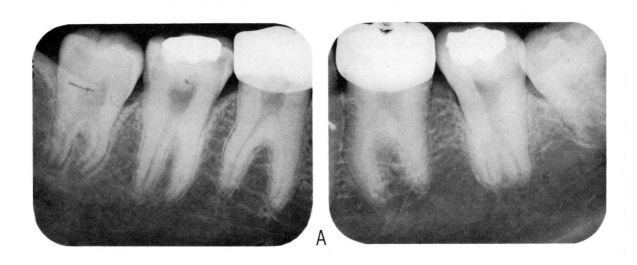

A

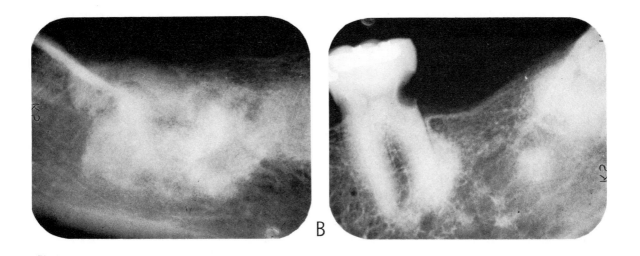

B

Plate 100     ACRYLIC BRIDGE; ACRYLIC DENTURE _____

**A.**     These two radiographs are from the same individual. The cuspids have been prepared for full-crown restorations, and a temporary acrylic bridge has been placed to maintain the space.

**B.**     A maxillary acrylic denture was left in the mouth when these bitewing radiographs were made.

Plate 100    ACRYLIC BRIDGE; ACRYLIC DENTURE

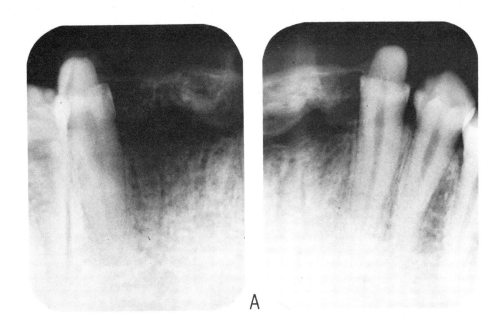

A

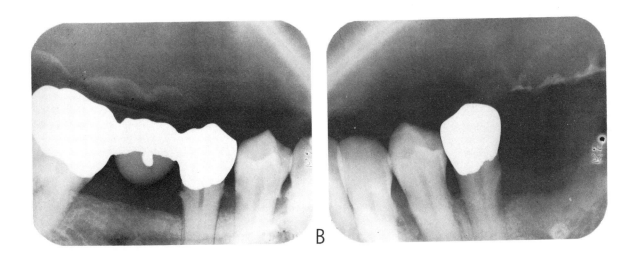

B

Plate 101    RADIOPAQUE MATERIALS; BIFID ROOTS _____

A.    The radiopaque objects lodged in the alveolus of the extracted second premolar are trapped silver alloy chips from restorations that were already in the first premolar. When the first premolar was prepared for its ceramic-fused-to-gold restoration, the silver alloy chips fell into the then unhealed alveolus.

B.    The patient was in an automobile accident. The large opaque object located apical to the teeth is a piece of leaded automobile glass.

C.    This premolar has an unusual bifid root formation.

D.    The cuspid also has an unusual bifid root formation.

Plate 101    RADIOPAQUE MATERIALS; BIFID ROOTS

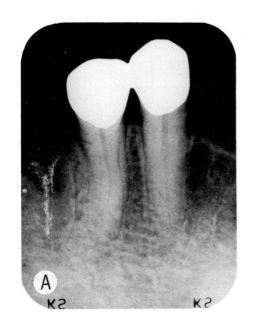

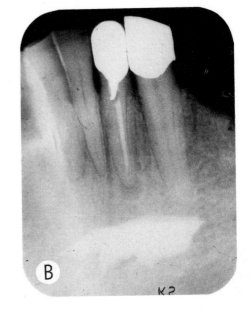

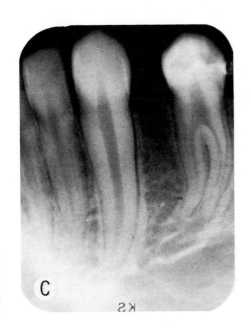

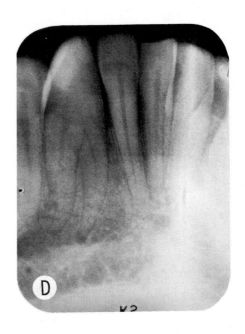

Plate 102    RESORPTION; OVERHANG; WOODEN HOLDERS; COTTON ROLLS _____

**A.**    The mesial root of the first molar has undergone much resorption. Note the mesial overhang of the restoration, which is causing the alveolar bone loss.

**B.**    The square, slightly opaque image at the top of the film is part of a wooden film holder. The visible image between the film holder and the alveolar ridge is a cotton roll.

**C.**    The third molar has apparently been impacted in bone for some time. It appears to be undergoing resorption. Note the mottled appearance of the crown.

**D.**    Between the wooden film holder and the alveolar ridge is the slightly opaque image of a cotton roll.

Plate 102    RESORPTION; OVERHANG; WOODEN HOLDERS; COTTON ROLLS

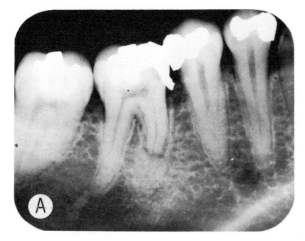

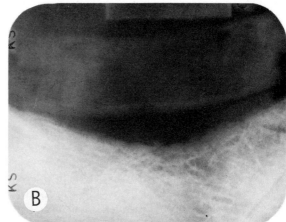

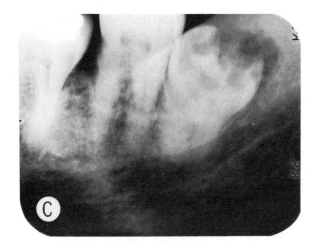

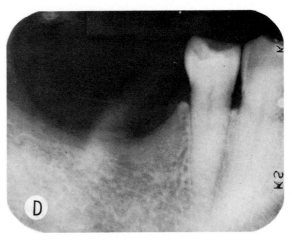

Plate 103     IMPACTION; CROSS-FIRE VIEW; LATERAL FACIAL VIEW _____

A.     An occlusal radiograph revealed the right central incisor impaction located near the nasal fossa.

B.     A cross-fire occlusal film was made in an attempt to locate the labial or palatal position of the tooth. As you see, this film does not show the tooth's location.

C.     This lateral facial film clearly shows the location of the tooth beneath the nasal fossa.

Plate 103    IMPACTION; CROSS-FIRE VIEW; LATERAL FACIAL VIEW

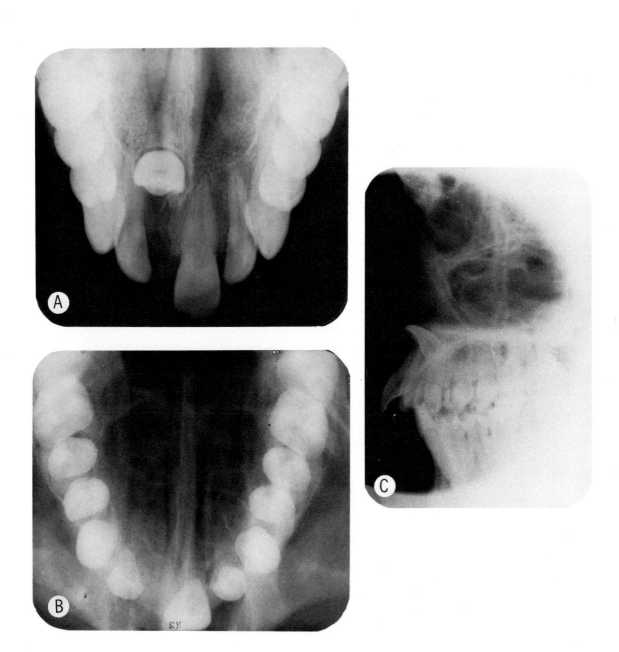

Plate 104     IMPACTION; CALCULUS; LANDMARKS; WORN GOLD CROWN _____

A.     The second primary molar remained in the maxillary arch. The second permanent premolar was not able to erupt properly and became impacted.

B.     This molar is covered with calculus.

C.     The maxillary tuberosity and the maxillary sinus are quite visible. An unusually long coronoid process is also visible.

D.     The dark spot seen on the crown of the first premolar is a worn surface of the gold crown.

Plate 104     IMPACTION; CALCULUS; LANDMARKS; WORN GOLD CROWN

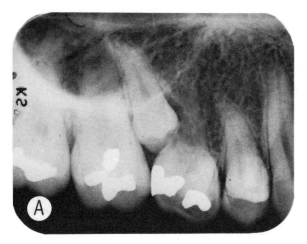

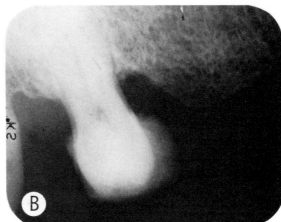

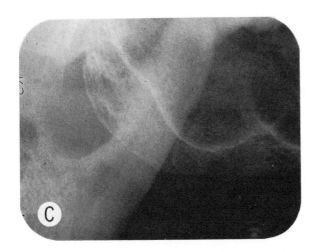

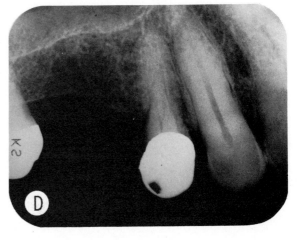

Plate 105     MANDIBULAR TORI ⸻

The large areas of radiopacity seen superimposed over the roots of these teeth are lingual mandibular tori.

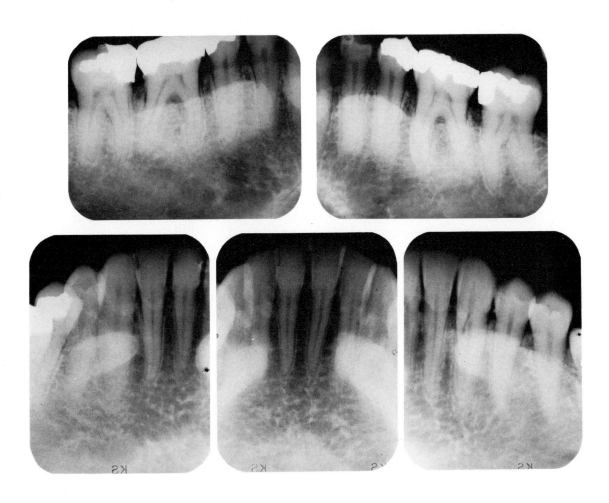

Plate 106    RESTORATIONS; WORN RESTORATIONS _____

A.    This was a functional three-unit gold bridge until the premolar abutment crown became so worn around the crown that the cervical portion of the crown collapsed in the position in which you now see it.

B.    In order to close the space between these two central incisors, the gold crown restoration was greatly over-contoured.

C.    This restoration was prepared in order to close the existing space between the two teeth. The metal covering the central incisor wore through.

D.    The pontic and distal abutment are all that remain of a three-unit bridge. The anterior bridge unit was lost some time before this radiograph was made.

Plate 106     RESTORATIONS; WORN RESTORATIONS

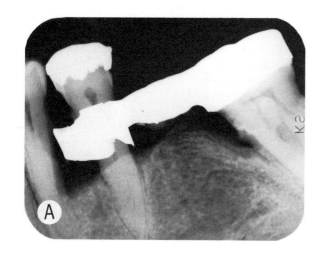

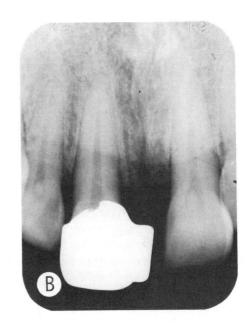

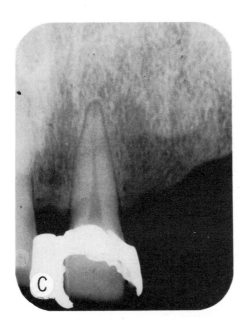

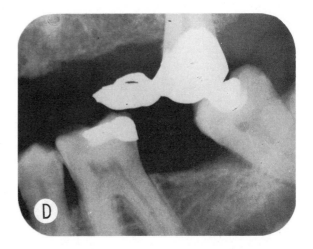

Plate 107    ROOT FRACTURE; MESIODENS; RESORPTION; BONE LOSS _____

**A.**    The right maxillary central incisor has a root fracture. Note that the apical third of the root canal appears calcified.

**B.**    The image seen between the maxillary central incisor roots is of a supernumerary tooth commonly called a mesiodens. The mesiodens appears to be resorbing, as indicated by the radiolucency.

**C.**    These teeth were endodontically treated. The general radiolucency of these teeth appears to indicate that they are undergoing resorption.

**D.**    Two poorly contoured crowns have been placed on these central incisors. There is a great deal of alveolar bone loss. Note also the calculus deposits on these teeth.

Plate 107    ROOT FRACTURE; MESIODENS; RESORPTION; BONE LOSS

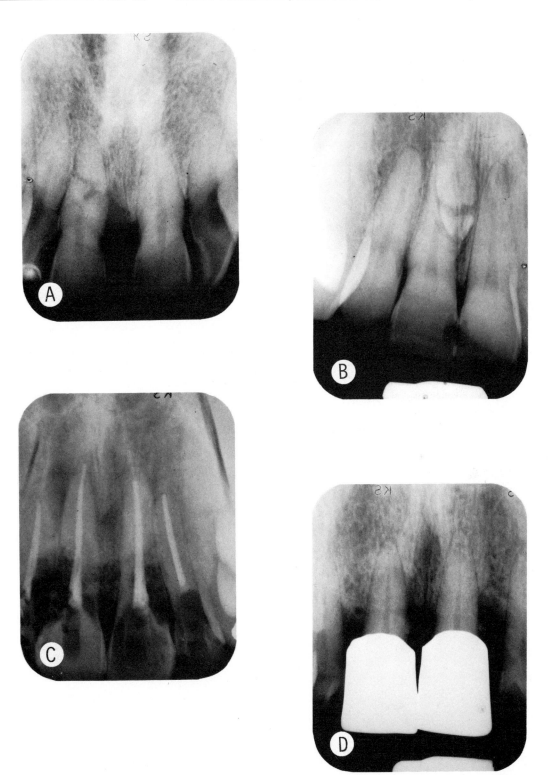

Plate 108     MAXILLARY SINUS RECESS; CARIES; ROOT REMNANTS _____

A.     The deep radiolucent spot in the maxillary sinus is called the maxillary
       sinus recess.
B.     The maxillary sinus recess is also seen in this film.
C.     Caries has taken its toll of these teeth. Multiple root remnants are seen
       in this film.
D.     Several root remnants are seen in the maxillary tuberosity. The coronoid
       process is just visible on the left of this film.

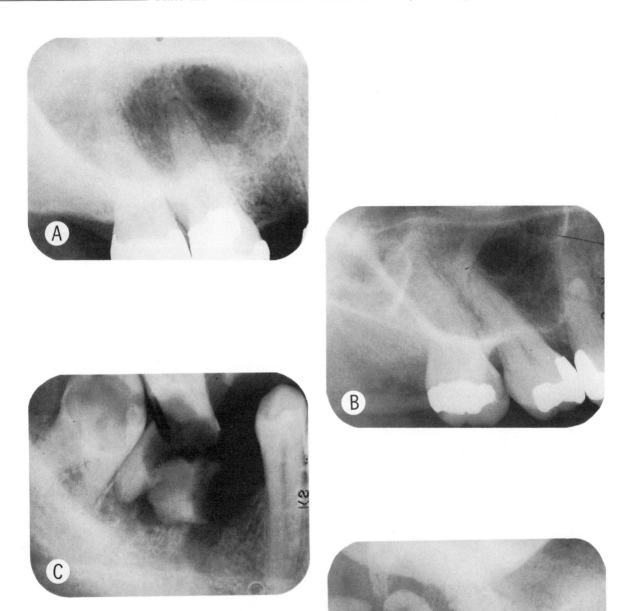

Plate 109    METALLIC ARTIFACT _____

**A.** This radiograph was made when the patient appeared at the dental clinic. The radiopaque mass superimposed over the root of the incisor does not appear to be a chemical artifact.

**B.** As it turns out, another film was placed under the patient's upper lip and this is the result. The radiopaque mass is still there, and it appears to be at the base of the anterior nasal spine. The patient stated that he had sustained an injury in an automobile accident several years earlier. This is either a piece of metal or leaded glass. Note the patient's lip.

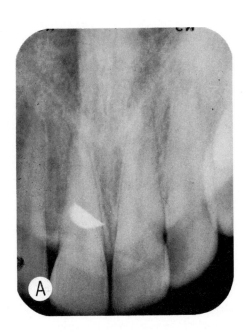

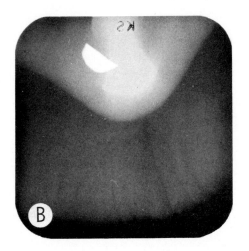

Plate 110    RESTORATIVE MATERIALS _____

**A.**   Reinforcing wires have been used in the restoring of the second pre-molar.

**B.**   Reinforcing wires have been used to restore the fractured mesial incisal edge of the central incisor.

**C.**   A vitreous carbon implant was used to replace the lost cuspid. Vitreous carbon material is radiolucent, but the gold post and core are radiopaque.

**D.**   These two central incisors were treated with gutta percha. The right incisor has a length of metal tubing that has been placed in the crown. The radiolucent areas seen in the tubing are small holes that have been placed in the tubing to assist with retention of resin restorative material.

Plate 110    RESTORATIVE MATERIALS

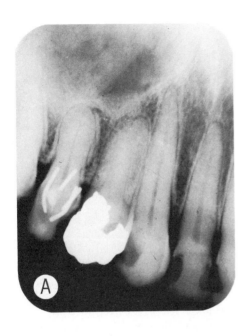

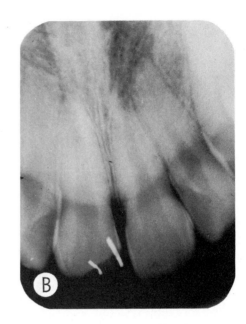

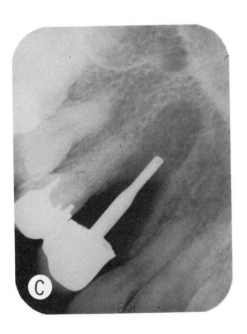

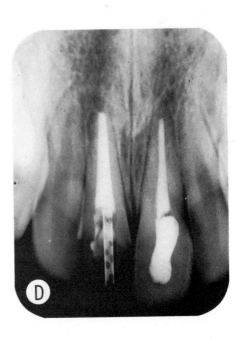

Plate 111    ROOT CARIES _____

**A.**    The cuspid does not appear to be as cariously involved as the other teeth. Cervical caries appears to circle the other teeth and is progressing along the root surfaces.

**B.**    Cervical caries is progressing along the tooth roots. The two vertical radiopaque lines were caused by bending or creasing of the radiographic film (the film emulsion apparently was not cracked).

**C.**    The large carious lesions have practically dissected what appears to be a cuspid tooth.

**D.**    The mesial root of the second molar and the distal root of the first molar show large carious lesions.

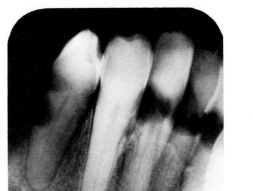

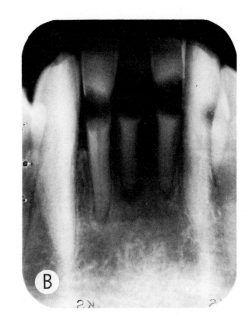

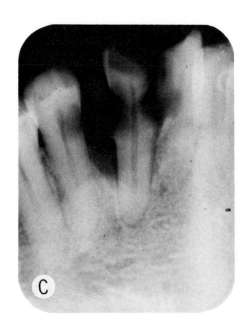

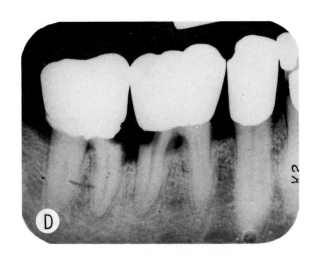

Plate 112     IMPACTION; CALCULUS; CYSTIC LESION

**A.**     The second premolar is impacted and appears to be undergoing resorption.

**B.**     Calculus shows up very well at the cervical aspect of these teeth.

**C.**     Equally clear evidence of calculus is seen in this radiograph.

**D.**     The second premolar will not be able to erupt normally. There is a lack of space between the first premolar and the first molar. The radiolucent area around the crown of the unerupted premolar might be a cyst; the tissue in this area should be checked by biopsy. The mesial aspect of the unerupted third molar can be seen.

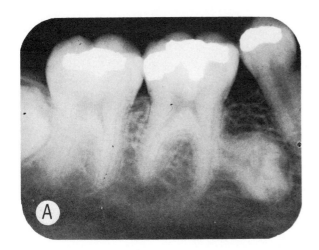

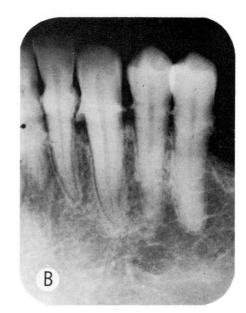

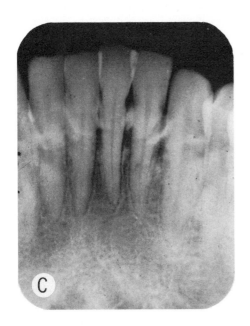

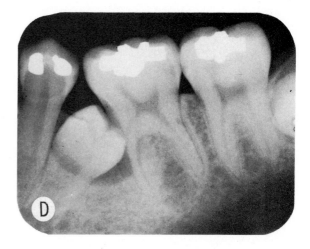

# *Index*